O R L

OXFORD RHEUMATOLOGY LIBRARY

Fibromyalgia Syndrome

► Except where otherwise stated, drug doses and recommendations are for the non-pregnant adult who is not breast-feeding.

ORL

OXFORD RHEUMATOLOGY LIBRARY

Fibromyalgia Syndrome

Dr Ernest Choy

Academic Department of Rheumatology,
King's College London,
Weston Education Centre,
London, UK

OXFORD
UNIVERSITY PRESS

OXFORD
UNIVERSITY PRESS

Great Clarendon Street, Oxford OX2 6DP

Oxford University Press is a department of the University of Oxford.
It furthers the University's objective of excellence in research, scholarship,
and education by publishing worldwide in

Oxford New York

Auckland Cape Town Dar es Salaam Hong Kong Karachi
Kuala Lumpur Madrid Melbourne Mexico City Nairobi
New Delhi Shanghai Taipei Toronto

With offices in

Argentina Austria Brazil Chile Czech Republic France Greece
Guatemala Hungary Italy Japan Poland Portugal Singapore
South Korea Switzerland Thailand Turkey Ukraine Vietnam

Oxford is a registered trade mark of Oxford University Press
in the UK and in certain other countries

Published in the United States
by Oxford University Press Inc., New York

First published 2009
UCB Pharma edition printed 2009

British Library Cataloguing in Publication Data

Data available

Library of Congress Cataloging in Publication Data

Data available

Typeset by Newgen Imaging Systems (P) Ltd., Chennai, India
Printed in Great Britain
on acid-free paper by
Ashford Colour Press Ltd., Gosport, Hants.

ISBN 978–0–19–957209–0

10 9 8 7 6 5 4 3 2 1

Contents

Preface

Fibromyalgia syndrome is characterized by chronic widespread pain. It is common, affecting 2–4% of the population. The prevalence has increased dramatically since 1990. The condition is not new but has been known by various names such as fibrositis or myofascial pain syndrome until 1990 when the American College of Rheumatology (ACR) published new classification criteria and first used the term fibromyalgia. The absence of an objective diagnostic test and overlap with other conditions often leads to significant delay in diagnosis. There is a general misconception that the condition is unresponsive to treatment yet there is evidence from published research to show that diagnosing and managing fibromyalgia positively leads to improvement of symptoms and quality of life. Indeed, healthcare utilization such as investigations, clinic visits, and referral to specialists decreases after diagnosis. Hence, it is vital for patients and clinicians that the condition is recognized and diagnosed early to avoid unnecessary anxiety and frustration.

The purpose of this short book is to provide a succinct and practical guide to help general practitioners and rheumatologists to diagnose and manage patients with fibromyalgia. This book will provide the reader with an essential understanding of the pathophysiology of pain in fibromyalgia, different subtypes of fibromyalgia, and pitfalls in diagnosis and management of this chronic condition.

Dr Ernest Choy, 2009

To Christina, Catrina, and Nicholas, for all their support and forbearance

Abbreviations

ACR	American College of Rheumatology
ACTH	adrenocorticotropic hormone
ARC	Arthritis Research Campaign
BDI	Beck Depression Inventory
cGMP	cyclic guanosine monophosphate
CGRP	calcitonin gene related peptide
CNS	central nervous system
CRH	corticotrophin-releasing hormone
CRP	C-reactive protein
CSF	cerebrospinal fluid
CSQ	Coping Strategies Questionnaire
ECG	electrocardiogram
ESR	erythrocyte sedimentation rate
EULAR	European League Against Rheumatism
FBC	full blood count
FEEL Study	Fibromyalgia & Epidemiology: European Large-Scale Study
FIQ	Fibromyalgia Impact Questionnaire
FM	fibromyalgia
fMRI	Functional Magnetic Resonance Imaging
FMS	fibromyalgia syndrome
GABA	gamma–aminobutyric acid
GMP	guanosine monophosphate
HADS	Hospital Anxiety Depression Scale
HAQ	Health Assessment Questionnaire
HPA	Hypothalamic–pituitary–adrenal axis
HRT	hormone replacement therapy
L5	lumbar spine
MINI	Mini International Neuropsychiatric Interview
NMDA	N-Methyl-d-Aspartate
NSAIDs	non-steroidal anti-inflammatory drugs

REM	rapid eye movement
RF	rheumatoid factor
SF-36	Short form-36
SNRIs	serotonin and norepinephrine re-uptake inhibitors
SSRIs	serotonin-selective-re-uptake inhibitors
STAI	State-Trait Anxiety Inventory
VAS	Visual Analogue Scale
VIP	Vasoactive intestinal peptide

Chapter 1

How to diagnose fibromyalgia syndrome

1

Key points

- Fibromyalgia syndrome (FMS) is characterized by chronic widespread pain and increased tenderness.
- Fatigue, unrefreshed sleep, depression, anxiety, and problems with cognition are common associated symptoms.
- Patients often complain of physical disability.
- American College of Rheumatology (ACR) criteria for FMS stipulates the presence of chronic widespread pain defined as pain in all four quadrants of the body, as well as in the axial skeleton for at least 3 months on a more-or-less continuous basis and the presence of at least 11 of 18 anatomically specific tender points.
- 'Red flag' symptoms are unexplained weight changes and fever.
- 'Red flag' signs are joint swelling, muscle weakness, abnormal gait, skin rashes, delayed tendon reflexes, and lymphadenopathies.

1.1 Introduction

Fibromyalgia syndrome (FMS) is not a new medical condition, although the term has only been used extensively since publication of the American College of Rheumatology (ACR) classification criteria in 1990. Numerous names, including muscular rheumatism, myalgia, interstitial fibrositis, myofascitis, and myofascial pain had been used to describe this condition since the 1800s. Although the term 'fibromyalgia syndrome' may not be ideal, it does not imply causation and describes the commonest symptom: chronic widespread pain. For the present, 'fibromyalgia syndrome' seems an appropriate compromise.

1.2 Clinical features: symptoms and signs

1.2.1 Pain

The universal feature in FMS is chronic widespread pain. This is defined as pain on both sides of the body as well as above and below the waist lasting for more than 3 months. Pain is predominantly axial and diffuse, but may affect any region and at different times be felt 'all over'. Characteristically, the patient complains 'I hurt all over all the time'. In some patients with FMS, there is a history of chronic local pain such as low back pain before developing more widespread pain.

Pain is variably described as burning, aching, or soreness. Although pain is present throughout the day without any significant diurnal variation, the location may change and the intensity varies. Physical activity often makes pain worse. However, many patients also complain of spontaneous pain without any obvious precipitating factor. Pain is often described as a chronic ache with occasional sharp spasm. Some patients describe their muscles to be tense and 'tied in knots'. Simple analgesics such as paracetamol or non-steroidal anti-inflammatory drugs (NSAIDs) are rarely effective.

One of the characteristic features of FMS is 'tenderness'. Patients often complain that even light touch or pressure is painful. Some patients complain that the slightest touch can make them recoil in pain.

Other painful conditions such as headache, migraine, non-cardiac chest pain, heartburn, dysmenorrhoea, and irritable bowel syndrome are common in patients with FMS.

Often patients complain of severe pain which is disabling. They cannot manage routine household chores especially shopping and cleaning. Those patients who are in employment often find it difficult coping with work.

1.2.2 Other major symptoms

Aside from pain, fatigue, non-restorative sleep, depression/anxiety, dyscognition, and disabilities are common in patients with FMS.

1.2.2.1 *Fatigue*

Fatigue is common in patients with FMS who are depressed, although patients without depression may still suffer from fatigue. Many patients rank fatigue as the second-most disabling symptom. It is often worse in the morning and early evening. Some patients associate fatigue with mild physical or mental exercise. Whilst the severity of fatigue varies, in general, it is less disabling than chronic fatigue syndrome. Nevertheless, in some patients, fatigue reduces their ability to perform daily chores and their quality of life.

1.2.2.2 *Non-restorative sleep*

Non-restorative sleep affects many patients with FMS. It is of pathogenic importance in some patients with fibromyalgia. This will be explained in more detail in Chapter 2. Patients often do not complain of sleeping disorder spontaneously. On enquiry, unrefreshing sleep occurs in about 65% of patients. Patients report poor sleep quality: they do not feel refreshed after a full night sleep, resulting in patients feeling tired, drained, and physically incapable of dealing with daily tasks. Many fibromyalgia sufferers find that they just cannot get adequate rest. Many feel drained and sleepy during the day. In some cases, patients complain of difficulty in getting to sleep or frequent wakefulness. The latter is particularly common in patients who suffer from frank sleep apnoea. Some patients linked sleep disturbance to the level of pain or fatigue.

Restless leg syndrome occurs in 20–40% of patients with FMS with unpleasant sensations in the lower limbs occurring at night, so much so that the limbs have to be moved in order to reduce the pain. It is linked to poor sleep quality and wakefulness.

In patients who complain of loud snoring and disturbances of breathing during the night, comorbid primary sleep disorders such as obstructive sleep apnoea syndrome should be suspected.

1.2.2.3 *Emotional: depression and anxiety*

Thirty to fifty per cent of patients with FMS suffer from significant depression or anxiety. In some patients, depression or anxiety may develop as a consequence of suffering from chronic widespread pain. However, in others, depression or anxiety predates the onset of chronic widespread pain, suggesting that the latter may result from emotion/mood disturbances. In these patients, the development of chronic widespread pain is often recognized at a time when their mood is low. It is useful to ask the patients directly whether they associate the chronic widespread pain with depression.

In general, it is useful to ask the patient whether they have any feeling of sadness, feelings of worthlessness or emptiness, lack of enjoyment in activities that once were pleasurable, poor appetite, and suicidal thoughts. The presence of the latter will need urgent psychiatric assessment.

Depression is often accompanied by fatigue, high pain score, and poor sleeping quality.

Anxiety often occurs with depression in patients with FMS; it can make existing symptoms, such as muscle pain and stiffness, even worse especially before the diagnosis is made and patients become increasingly concerned and frustrated with their symptoms. In severe cases, patients may complain of panic attacks. Symptoms often associated with anxiety include dizziness, excessive sweating, shortness of breath, dysphagia, palpitation, and tingling sensations.

1.2.2.4 *Dyscognition*

Patients with FMS often report problems with cognition. Symptoms include problems with memory; inability to concentrate and focus on tasks; trouble in retaining new information; and difficulties with doing mental arithmetic, problem solving, and learning new tasks. In the United States, the term 'Fibrofog' has been used to describe this problem in cognition because sufferers often describe a feeling of being in a fog. They are often episodic and typically last for a few days, although, in some cases, it may be more prolonged.

Dyscognition often leads to difficulty at work and problem in carrying out normal household chores. It has a major impact on quality of life and functionality, especially in patients whose work is mentally demanding. It is a major contributor of frustration and psychosocial stress.

1.2.2.5 *Functional disability*

Most patients with FMS have difficulties coping with work and household chores. Both physical and mental difficulties contribute to functional disability and reduction in quality of life, including work, home, and social relationships, which in turn increases psychosocial stress. Assessing these in the medical history is important for formulating a management plan.

1.2.3 **Other symptoms**

In addition to pain and major symptoms, individuals with FMS may suffer from a myriad of other symptoms. Although the physiological basis of these symptoms remains incompletely understood, increasing evidence implicates psychosocial stress and dysfunction of the autonomic nervous system in the pathophysiology.

Most patients complain of morning stiffness of variable duration. Many patients complain of tissues feeling swollen as well as numbness and tingling in upper and lower limbs, although objective evidence is often lacking.

Chronic headaches, chest pain, shortness of breath, and palpitations are common. These are often the result of anxiety, but a careful cardiovascular evaluation should be carried out to exclude serious cardiac illnesses.

Gastrointestinal symptoms such as nausea, vomiting, bloating, abdominal pain, diarrhoea, and constipation are common and often related to irritable bowel syndrome.

Uro-gynaecological symptoms including urgency, frequency, incontinence, pelvic pain, and dysmenorrhoea are also common.

Unexplained weight loss or gain and fever are 'red flag' symptoms and strongly suggest alternative diagnoses.

1.3 Clinical features: physical examination

The goal of the physical examination is to confirm diagnosis and rule out other systemic diseases. Hence, a full medical examination is important. In patients with FMS, clinical findings are usually unremarkable. Examine the patient's gait, range of joint movement, and deformities. Objective evidence of muscle weakness, synovitis, heart murmur, slow tendon reflexes, or other neurological abnormality would strongly suggest other diseases such as hypothyroidism and myopathies which require further detailed investigation. Osteoarthritis and tendonitis are common incidental findings.

1.3.1 Tender points and tenderness: hyperalgesia and allodynia

The presence of multiple hyperalgesic tender points is a typical finding in FMS. When sufficient pressure/stimulus is applied over any part of our body, pain is experienced. This is normal nocioception. Patients with FMS have reduced pressure pain threshold, experiencing pain with normally innocuous pressure: allodynia. When noxious stimulus or pressure is applied, patients with FM experience more severe pain than normal individuals: hyperalgesia. A more detailed explanation of the pathophysiology of hyperalgesia and allodynia is given in Chapter 3. Elicit these tender points as important in establishing the diagnosis of FMS.

1.4 ACR classification criteria for FMS

Before 1990, no guidelines for diagnosing fibromyalgia existed. To facilitate research to ensure similar patient cohorts are recruited, the ACR published the 'classification criteria' for the diagnosis of FMS. It stipulates two basic requirements:

1. First, the presence of chronic widespread pain defined as pain in all four quadrants of the body, as well as in the axial skeleton for at least 3 months on a more-or-less continuous basis.
2. Second, the presence of at least 11 of 18 anatomically specific tender points. They include nine sites bilaterally: occiput, low cervical, supraspinatus, trapezius, second rib, lateral epicondyle, gluteal, greater trochanter, and medial knee.

These naturally occurring sites are uncomfortable to firm digital pressure in normal individuals, but in FMS similar pressure elicits marked tenderness and often a wince/withdrawal response. The thumb should be used to apply pressure to the site. A tender point hurts only at the area where pressure (enough to cause the examiner's nail bed to blanch, or about 4kg) is applied. These must be reported as 'painful' not just 'tender' (Figure 1.1).

Figure 1.1 American College for Rheumatology (ACR) classification criteria for FM: tender point sites

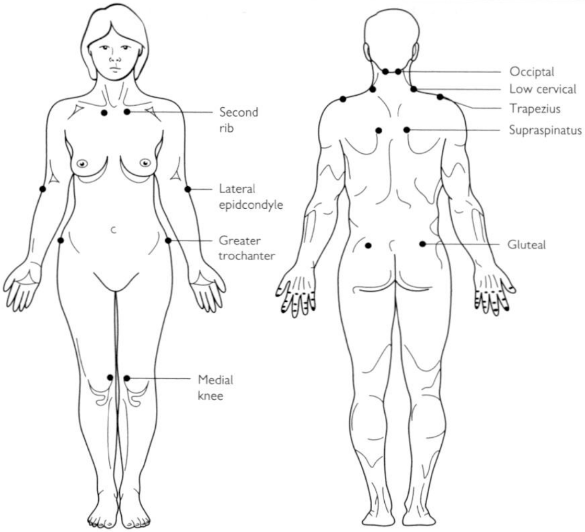

ACR classification criteria for FM: tender point sites are listed in Table 1.1.

Table 1.1 American College of Rheumatology classification criteria for fibromyalgia: tender point sites

Bilateral Sites	Anatomical Location
1. Occiput	At the nuchal ridge, laterally one-thumb width to the insertion of the suboccipital muscle to the occiput
2. Low cervical	At the fifth through seventh intertransverse spaces of the cervical spine
3. Supraspinatus	At the craniomedial border of the scapula at the origin of the supraspinatus
4. Trapezius	At the upper border of the shoulder in the trapezius muscle midway from the neck to the shoulder joint
5. Second rib	In the pectoral muscle at the second costochondral junctions
6. Lateral epicondyle	Approximately three-finger breadths (2cm) below the lateral epicondyle
7. Gluteal	In the upper outer quadrant of the gluteus medius
8. Greater trochanter	Just posterior to the prominence of the greater trochanter at the piriformis insertion
9. Medial knee	At the medial fat pad proximal to the joint line

Figure 1.1 is reproduced with permission from Wolfe F, Smythe HA, Yunus MB, *et al*. The American College of Rheumatology 1990 criteria for the classification of fibromyalgia. Report of the Multicenter Criteria Committee. *Arthritis Rheum*, 1990; **33**: 160–72.

1.5 Differential diagnoses

The list of differential diagnoses includes diseases which may cause widespread pain and weakness:

- Primary generalized osteoarthritis
- Polymyalgia rheumatica
- Rheumatoid arthritis
- Autoimmune connective tissue diseases such as systemic lupus erythematosus and inflammatory muscle diseases
- Myopathies
- Hypothyroidism
- Malignancies.

Sometimes FMS may occur concomitantly with osteoarthritis, rheumatoid arthritis, hypothyroidism, and autoimmune connective tissue diseases. In such cases, the diagnosis of FMS should be considered when the severity of pain does not correlate with disease activity.

The following are a list of 'red flag' symptoms and signs suggestive of alternative diagnosis:

Symptoms:

1. Significant changes in weight
2. Fever
3. Sleep apnoea (loud and excessive snoring).

Signs:

1. Joint swelling
2. Muscle weakness
3. Abnormal gait
4. Skin rashes
5. Delayed tendon reflexes
6. Lymphadenopathy
7. Focal neurological signs.

1.6 Investigations

Laboratory and radiological investigations in FMS are used to exclude differential diagnoses.

List of blood tests should include

1. Full blood count
2. Erythrocyte sedimentation rate
3. Biochemistries
4. Liver function test
5. Thyroid function test

6. Muscle enzymes (creatine phosphokinases)
7. Rheumatoid factor and auto-antibodies tests should be performed especially if rheumatoid arthritis or autoimmune connective tissue diseases are suspected. However, false positive rate is significant.

Radiological examination is generally unnecessary.

Muscle weakness or abnormal neurological examination may require nerve conduction study and electromyography.

1.7 Associated conditions

In the past, the term 'secondary fibromyalgia' has been applied when FM superimposes upon pre-existing painful conditions such as osteoarthritis or rheumatoid arthritis. When it affects individuals without other chronic painful conditions, it is referred to as 'primary fibromyalgia'. However, the ACR classification criteria do not separate primary and secondary fibromyalgia.

1.8 Overlap with somatization

FMS shares many common features with, and often co-exists with, other syndromes such as irritable bowel syndrome, chronic fatigue syndrome, and dysmenorrhagia, leading to the suggestion that it is part of a spectrum of disorders characterized by somatization. There is also obvious overlap in symptoms and impaired function between FMS, anxiety, and depression. Indeed, patients with FMS often score highly on anxiety and depression questionnaires. However, many patients with FMS are not depressed and clinical response to antidepressant is often independent to changes in mood.

1.9 Controversy

The diagnosis of FMS has been disputed by some clinicians. They have argued that FMS is not a distinct disease entity, and labelling patients with FMS would encourage chronic illness state and increase healthcare utilization. The overlap with somatization was used to support their argument.

However, it is clear the patient problem of FMS has been recognized for many years. Medicine has a bias towards a pathological explanation of 'disease', and these conditions have often been considered expressions of psychological disturbance of little medical interest. Such symptoms and disability, however, are real, not fabricated or imagined, and reflect 'functional' rather than 'pathological' abnormality. Recently, with advances in neuroimaging, especially with functional magnetic resonance imaging (fMRI) scan, such functional abnormality can be objectively assessed and demonstrated in FMS. The condition may not be homogeneous in expression, but this is no different from many medical conditions such as osteoarthritis and rheumatoid arthritis. Research in the United Kingdom has shown that it is an increasing healthcare burden, but using the diagnosis of fibromyalgia constructively reduces healthcare utilization. Furthermore, effective treatments are available. More detailed explanation will be given in later chapters of this book. Hence, it is a mistake to ignore FMS as a medical problem.

1.10 Summary

Recent research showed that the diagnosis is often delayed for 5 years and many unnecessary referral and investigations are performed prior to the diagnosis. Prompt recognition and diagnosis are important to both patients and healthcare state. The ACR has established classification criteria which are simple to apply in routine clinical setting for the diagnosis of FMS.

Useful practical hints

- Ask about site, duration, onset, and severity of pain.
- Ask patients whether they feel tired all the time.
- Ask the patients whether they sleep well and whether they feel refreshed in the morning.
- Ask patients whether they feel depressed, anxious, or feel pressurized/stressed at home and at work. In patients with depression, ask whether they have any suicidal thoughts. The presence of the latter will need urgent psychiatric assessment.
- Ask patients whether they have any problem with memory, or difficulties with concentration, problem-solving, and learning new tasks.
- Ask about the impact of illness on daily life, work, and social relationships.
- Remember to ask the 'red flag' symptoms: unexplained weight changes and fever.
- Conduct general medical examination and assess the number of FM tender points.
- Remember the red flag signs: joint swelling, muscle weakness, abnormal gait, skin rashes, delayed tendon reflexes, and lymphadenopathies.

Suggested reading

Bennett RM (1989). Confounding features of the fibromyalgia syndrome: a current perspective of differential diagnosis. *Journal of Rheumatology Supplement*, Nov; **19**: 58–61.

Clauw DJ and Crofford LJ (2003). Chronic widespread pain and fibromyalgia: what we know, and what we need to know. *Best Practice and Research Clinical Rheumatology*, Aug; **17**(4): 685–701.

Goldenberg DL (1987). Fibromyalgia syndrome. An emerging but controversial condition. *Journal of American Medical Association,* **257**: 2782–7.

Goldenberg DL (1989). Psychiatric and psychologic aspects of fibromyalgia syndrome. *Rheumatic Disease Clinics of North America*, **15**: 105–14.

Mease P (2005). Fibromyalgia syndrome: review of clinical presentation, pathogenesis, outcome measures, and treatment. *Journal of Rheumatology Supplement*, **75**: 6–21.

Wolfe F, Smythe HA, Yunus MB, *et al.* (1990). The American College of Rheumatology 1990 criteria for the classification of fibromyalgia. *Arthritis and Rheumatism*, **33**: 160–72.

Chapter 2

Epidemiology and healthcare burden of fibromyalgia syndrome

Key points

- Fibromyalgia syndrome (FMS) is common, affecting 2% of the population.
- It is more common in women than in men, with a gender ratio of 7:1.
- Physical function and quality of life is often reduced. Most patients have chronic disease. Spontaneous remission is uncommon.
- Medical cost is high up to 10 years prior to diagnosis. Societal cost of FMS due to reduced productivity is high. Constructive diagnosis can reduce healthcare cost.

2.1 History of fibromyalgia syndrome (FMS)

The first accurate description of fibromyalgia symptoms appeared in the mid-1800s. In 1850, Froriep reported that patients with 'rheumatism' had hard places in their muscles which were painful to pressure. The term 'fibrositis' was introduced by Gowers in 1904, although he actually described regional pain syndromes including sensitivity to touch in association with fatigue and sleep disturbances in the absence of any signs of local or systemic inflammation. In the 1930s, Lewis and Kellgren injected hypertonic saline into deep muscle tissue and induced referred muscle pain. The distribution of pain referral patterns was uniform and differed from dermatomal patterns. During the next half-century, fibrositis, as it was then called, was considered by some to be a common cause of muscular pain, by others to be a manifestation of 'tension' or 'psychogenic rheumatism', and by the rheumatology community in general to be a non-entity.

Smythe and Moldofsky introduced the current concept of FMS in the 1970s through studies in which they described that certain anatomic locations were more tender in patients with FMS than in controls. These 'tender points' were often identical to those most tender in regional pain conditions such as 'tennis elbow', 'costochondritis', and cervical strain syndromes. Importantly, they first showed that patients with FMS had a stage 4 sleep disturbance, and that experimental selective stage 4 disturbance produced the symptoms and muscle tenderness consistent with FMS in healthy volunteers.

Subsequently, the diagnostic utility of tender points was verified by a series of studies in the 1980s from different researchers. Many diagnostic criteria were developed, based on presence of pain, tender points, and other symptoms and the exclusion of other rheumatic or systemic diseases. However, many observers have noted the concomitant occurrence of FMS with chronic painful rheumatic disease. This led to the introduction of the concept of primary and secondary FMS. Over the years, authors debated the optimal number of tender points, as well as the relevance of the concept of primary and secondary fibromyalgia. In 1990, the American College of Rheumatology (ACR) criteria for the classification of fibromyalgia was published by a North American multicentre criteria committee. This was developed by assessing 293 patients with FMS and 265 controls. They were interviewed and examined by trained, blinded assessors. Controls were matched for age and sex and all had a rheumatic disorder that could be easily confused with fibromyalgia, such as 'possible' rheumatoid arthritis. The combination of widespread pain, defined as bilateral, above and below the waist, and axial, and at least 11 of 18 specified tender points, yielded a sensitivity of 88.4% and a specificity of 81.1%. There were no significant differences in patients considered to have primary/concomitant versus secondary fibromyalgia, and for classification purposes such distinctions were to be discarded. No exclusions were made for laboratory or radiographic findings. The ACR classification criteria was developed to facilitate research so that a homogeneous population of patients can be studied, allowing different studies to be pooled or compared. Although it was not designed primarily as diagnostic criteria, it is now widely used as such in routine clinical practice.

2.2 Epidemiology

Using the ACR classification criteria, the prevalence of FMS in the general population ranges from 0.5% to 4%. The prevalence of FMS in medical outpatient clinics is much higher than in the general population and ranged from 10% to 16% in rheumatology outpatient clinics. It can affect children as well as adults.

Gender: FMS is 3–7 times more common in women than in men. The gender ratio tends to be higher in hospital compared with general population studies.

Age: FMS may be diagnosed in individuals of all ages. Symptoms usually arise in those aged 20–55 years, but the condition may occur in childhood. In the ACR 1990 classification criteria study, the mean age was 49 years, with 89% of patients being female. This prevalence increased with age, reaching 7% in women of age 60–80 years.

Ethnicity: No racial predilection exists in FMS. Researchers have reported the condition in all ethnic groups and cultures. In the United States, 93% were Caucasian, 5% Hispanic, and 1% Black. Comparison between patients with FMS has been made in Europe and the United States. No significant difference in manifestation was found.

2.2.1 Global prevalence in the general population

FMS is prevalent in all countries, unrelated to the level of industrialization and local culture. Prior to the publication of the ACR criteria, estimates of the prevalence of FMS varied from 1% to 2% in population survey. Since the ACR criteria were published, a number of studies have assessed point prevalence of FMS by screening questionnaire followed by detail assessment. In Canada, an epidemiological study found that the point prevalence of ACR-defined FMS in the general population was 3%. A similar population-based epidemiological study in Europe—the FEEL study (Fibromyalgia & Epidemiology: European large-scale survey)—found that a point prevalence of possible FMS in France and Portugal was 7.4% and 10.45%, respectively.

2.2.2 Population versus clinical practice

Whilst population point prevalence of FMS is approximately 2%, FM accounts for 2.1% attendance in family practice clinic, 5.7% in a general medical clinic, 5–8% in a hospital setting, and 14–20% in a rheumatology clinic.

2.2.3 Risk factors

Many studies have shown that psychological conditions such as somatization, having a mental disorder, presence of psychological distress, major depression, panic disorder, and familial major mood disorder are risk factors for developing FMS. Previous trauma and socio-cultural factors such as less education, low level of income, being divorced, being disabled, being an immigrant, smoking, and lower social class have all been implicated but definitive evidence of causation is lacking.

A number of studies have suggested that genetic factors play an important role in the development of FMS. Twenty-eight per cent of offspring of mothers with FM suffer from chronic widespread pain.

One case controlled study also found strongly familial aggregation of FM. The risk of suffering from FMS in a relative of a proband with FM was increased eightfold when compared with probands of rheumatoid arthritis. A study comparing the prevalence of chronic widespread pain in monozygotic and dizygotic twins found that genetic factors accounted for 50% of the total variance. This provides persuasive evidence supporting the importance of genetic factor in the pathogenesis of FMS.

A number of candidate genes have been suggested which include polymorphisms of genes in the serotonergic, catecholaminergic, and dopaminergic systems. Overall, it is highly likely that polygenetic factors may act in concert with environmental factors in the development of FMS.

2.2.4 **Drawback of ACR classification criteria**

When the ACR classification criteria were developed, it was thought that there may be local pathologies at the sites of tender points. However, recent research has shown that tenderness is widespread in FMS and can be elicited in many parts of the body. The pathophysiology of this increased tenderness will be explained in Chapter 3. The stipulated tender point criteria not only misrepresents the pathophysiology of the condition but also more importantly affects the epidemiology of the condition.

Furthermore, the number of tender point count correlates more highly with psychological distress than with tenderness/pressure pain threshold as measured by dolorimetry. The number of tender points is also influenced by gender. Even in healthy individuals, women are more likely to have a higher number of tender points than men. Research has shown that women are 11 times more likely than men to fulfil the ACR criteria for having at least 11 tender points. This results in the condition being under-diagnosed and its prevalence under-estimated in men.

A recent study comparing diagnosis of FMS based on ACR criteria with clinical finding or survey found that the agreement was only moderate. It also showed that the cut-off of 11 tender points was insensitive for diagnosis of FMS. Using six tender points as a cut-off was more sensitive without losing specificity.

The problem with ACR classification criteria led to several epidemiological studies using chronic widespread pain as a definition to study this condition in the community. Chronic widespread pain is common. In developed countries, the prevalence of chronic widespread pain is 7–13% based on population studies in the United Kingdom, Sweden, and North America. Chronic regional pain such as low back pain affects 20–25% of the population. Both conditions are more common in women with a female to male ratio of 1:5. However, chronic widespread pain is only modestly associated with distress, and distress is only weakly associated with the subsequent development of chronic widespread pain. Many people with chronic widespread pain do not have or subsequently develop distress or depression.

2.2.5 Summary of epidemiology

Both chronic widespread pain and FM are very common. The prevalence of chronic widespread pain in the community is higher than FMS. In the community, many patients fulfil the ACR classification criteria without the diagnosis being made. Hence the diagnosis does not create the syndrome, but patients with FMS are prevalent in the community. FMS may represent a continuum of chronic widespread pain in the population. The impression of high female-to-male ratio of FMS may be due to the stipulated tender point count threshold by the ACR classification criteria which tends to bias against men. FMS is now the second or the third most common disorder that rheumatolgists evaluate and treat. Rheumatologists may find that approximately 10–20% of their patients have FMS.

The perception of many clinicians associating FMS with women who have high levels of psychological stress owes much to the ACR classification criteria stipulation for at least 11 tender points, and many studies have recruited patients with FMS from hospital-based outpatient clinics where psychological and psychiatric comorbidities are much higher than in the community.

2.3 Prognosis

In general, FMS is neither progressive nor fatal. Most studies show that treatment can significantly improve symptoms, function, and quality of life in the short term. In general, children with FMS tend to have better outlooks than adults do. Although these studies provide optimism for better outcomes in FMS, prospective long-term cohort studies based in tertiary hospitals in North America and Europe found no significant change in prognosis over a 6- to 8-year period. Severity of pain, fatigue, disability, and quality of life remained unchanged. Furthermore, they found little improvement in health status, health service utilization, and costs, with approximately 25% of patients with FMS receiving disability or other compensation payments. Health status in patients with FMS is at least as poor, if not worse than those with other musculoskeletal diseases, such as rheumatoid arthritis. Predictors of poor outcome include significant life crisis or severe disability. However, patients with FMS in the community may have milder condition and better prognosis than those seen in specialist centres. Granges *et al.* reported a 24% remission rate after 2 years of patients. Other studies found 25–35% of patients with FMS report improvement in pain over time, although it is rare for symptoms to subside completely.

It is important for patients to realize that complete remission is rare and there is no simple cure for FMS. They should be encouraged to have a positive attitude and develop better coping strategies with the help of healthcare professionals. Studies have shown that a good outcome is related to having a positive attitude and an effective coping strategy. Resolution of ongoing stress and promotion of the patient's self-efficacy for control of pain are of pivotal importance in maintaining long-term improvement. A notable example is the benefit of regular exercise. One study suggested that patients with FMS who exercise regularly over a period of 4 years have a better outcome. With the lack of a universal panacea, a multidisciplinary approach will be necessary to manage FMS especially for patients with more severe or a wide range of symptoms.

2.4 Quality of life

FMS varies significantly in severity. However, quality of life is generally reduced. Both impaired physical function and emotional impact adversely affect the quality of life of patients with FMS. Approximately 50% of all patients have difficulty with routine daily activities, while 30–40% have to stop work or change their employment. The lack of support from family, friends, and healthcare system may further compound the problem. Some have compared the social, emotional, economic, and functional effect of FMS on an individual's life with the effects of rheumatoid arthritis. On a scale of 1–10 (0 = lowest and 10 = highest), the average 'present quality of life' score for patients with FMS was 4.8. Although, standard, generic human-related quality of life instruments may be insensitive to capture quality-of-life issues for many people with FMS.

2.4.1 Physical function

Patients with FMS often find it difficult to perform daily activities. Almost half the patients reported some disability. Many patients complain of stiffness in the morning and need more time to get started. Often they struggle with tasks which require sustained or repetitive physical effort. This is often aggravated by cold weather.

Quality of life, measured by Medical Outcomes Study Short Form-36 Health Survey, in patients with FMS has been compared with rheumatoid arthritis and healthy individuals. Physical functioning, physical role, social functioning, bodily pain, general health, vitality, emotional role, and mental health scores were significantly lower in rheumatoid arthritis and FMS patients than in control subjects. Patients with FMS had significantly lower mental health scores than rheumatoid patients. Indeed, psychological factors/mental health seem to play a pronounced disabling role in FMS.

2.4.2 **Mental health/psychological stress**

One study compared the quality of life and general health status of 98 patients with FMS with 48 healthy volunteers using the Nottingham Health Profile. Patients with FMS have significantly higher Nottingham Health Profile scores indicative of poorer general health status. Nottingham Health Profile scores correlated with disease activity as measured by Tender Point Count, Fibromyalgia Impact Questionnaire (FIQ), and Health Assessment Questionnaire score. Patients with depression tend to have a higher Nottingham Health Profile score. This suggests an important relationship between pain, depression, and quality-of-life scales in patients with FMS. Moreover, Nottingham Health Profile score correlated with disease duration, suggesting that chronicity may adversely impact general health and quality of life.

A telephone survey in Spain based on patients with FMS attending a university hospital found them to have an average FIQ score of 63.6. Poor quality of life correlated with having a larger number of children, being tired and being in a depressed mood, reference to repercussion on the family environment, and a lower self-rated health. Importantly, those consulted more specialists before the diagnosis of FMS was associated with a poor quality of life.

2.4.3 **Sleep disturbance and quality of life**

A study in over 100 patients with FMS found that sleep quality was significantly predictive of pain, fatigue, and social functioning. Therefore, interventions designed to improve sleep quality may help to restore health-related quality of life in FMS.

2.4.4 **Risk of negative behaviours**

Severity of pain, poor emotional health, and sleep disturbances either alone or in combination may lead to excessive self-medication and overuse of sleeping pills, alcohol, drugs, or caffeine. A study in 2001 found a higher incidence of violent deaths, including suicide and accidents, among people with chronic widespread pain.

Quality of life is poor in patients with FMS; not surprisingly, patients with significant mood involvement fare worse, given the association between worse outcome and prior consultation before diagnosis and chronicity. Prompt diagnosis and positive management may prevent the development of a vicious cycle leading to the condition spiralling out of control.

2.5 Healthcare burden

In the United States, the annual direct healthcare cost of FMS in 1996 was $2274 per patient. Hospitalization and day care services were the main expenditures. Data from the National Center for Chronic Disease Prevention and Health Promotion showed that in 1997, 7440 hospitalizations were related to FMS. It accounts for 2.2 million ambulatory care visits, 1.8 million physician office visits, 266 000 Emergency Department visits, and 187 000 Outpatient Department visits. The average patient makes ten primary care appointments per year and is hospitalized on average once every 3 years. The cost of management of FMS in primary care clinics is high because of the diagnostic tests and treatment. Patients with FMS were more likely to be referred to hospital specialists and had diagnostic procedures. Confronted by such statistics, the Chief Medical Officer in the United Kingdom wrote to all the doctors in the United Kingdom emphasizing the healthcare burden of chronic widespread pain, and urging that more research and information are essential to address the problem and improve outcome.

When compared to other chronic diseases such as diabetes mellitus and hypertension, patients with FMS consume healthcare resources to a similar extent, but the latter receive far less attention from the healthcare system. Greater awareness of this disorder can improve management and facilitate planning of healthcare resources, thus improving quality of care. Indeed, a recent study in the United Kingdom supports such premise. Based on the United Kingdom General Practice Research Database, a large database covering 5 million patients found that healthcare utilization in patients with FMS was already very high compared with disease controls, matched on diagnosis date, gender, and age, up to 10 years prior to diagnosis. Increase in cost was due to a higher rate of visits, prescriptions, and diagnostic tests. Patients with FMS averaged 25 visits and 11 prescriptions per year compared with 12 visits and 4.5 prescriptions per year in controls. Following the diagnosis of FM, the rate of consultations stabilized and then declined to 13 per 100 patient per year by 4 years post diagnosis (Figure 2.1a). Overall rates of referrals and tests were significantly higher in FM cases compared with controls. Following the FMS diagnosis, referral rates declined considerably and the incidence of tests appeared to stabilize (Figure 2.1b). Rheumatology referrals dropped to near-control levels by 4 years following the diagnosis. This is evidence that the diagnosis of FM, which is made mainly by rheumatologists in the United Kingdom, may be used constructively in the management of FMS.

Figure 2.1 The impact of diagnosis of FMS on healthcare cost: (a) Total number of clinic visits and (b) Number of diagnostic tests

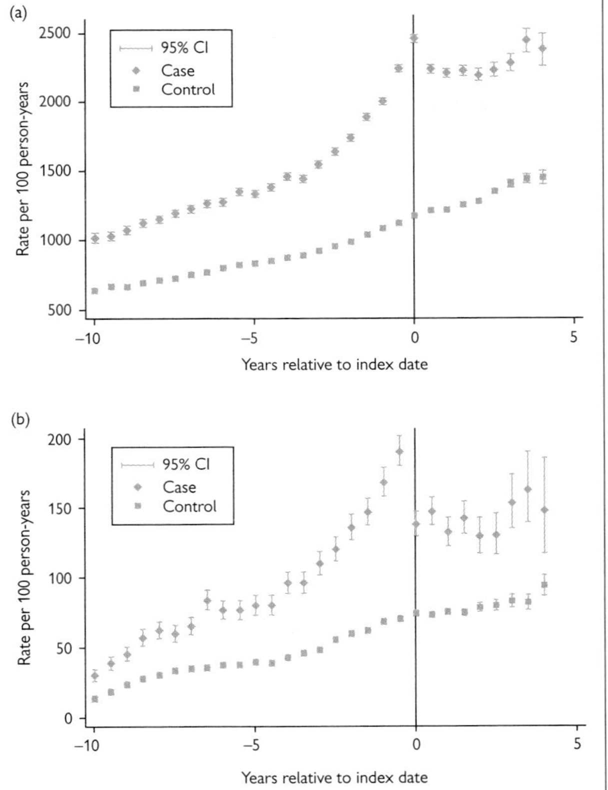

Figures 2.1 (a) & (b) reproduced from Hughes G, Martinez C, Myon E, et al. (2006). The impact of a diagnosis of fibromyalgia on health care resource use by primary care patients in the UK: an observational study based on clinical practice. Arthritis & Rheumatism, Jan; **54**(1): 177–83.

2.6 Social cost

The cost of FM to both the individual and to society is huge. Approximately one-third of patients with FMS have to adapt their work, shorten their workdays or workweeks, or do both to keep their jobs. Others have to change jobs that are less demanding physically and mentally. This change often leads to decreased income and increased financial burdens. The hidden costs of disability and comorbidities greatly increase the true burden of FMS. A study in Europe showed that average annual disease-related total societal cost for FMS was €7813 per patient. In the United States, the indirect medical cost in 1997 amounts to $3671. A survey in the United States found that 42% of patients with FMS were employed and 28% were homemakers. The total annual costs for FMS claimants were more than twice as high as the costs for the typical insurance beneficiary. The prevalence of disability was twice as high among FMS employees as overall employees. For every dollar spent on FMS-specific claims, employers spent about $60–140 on additional direct and indirect costs. Twenty to thirty per cent of patients were receiving disability payment, with 16% receiving Social Security benefits. The estimated overall annual cost of FMS to the economy in the United States is over $9 billion. It accounts for a loss of 1–2% of the nation's overall productivity.

Although the financial cost of FMS is high, the personal/emotional cost to patients, their families, and friends is staggering. Relationships are strained at best and many times are destroyed by this illness.

2.7 Summary

FMS is common but under-recognized. Physical disability, sleep, and mood disturbances result in poor quality of life. The direct and indirect medical costs of FMS are high. Whilst the ACR criteria are not perfect, applying it constructively in routine clinical setting can reduce healthcare burden of this chronic debilitating condition.

Suggested reading

Gallagher AM, Thomas JM, Hamilton WT, White PD (2004). Incidence of fatigue symptoms and diagnoses presenting in UK primary care from 1990 to 2001. *Journal of the Royal Society of Medicine*, **97**: 571–5.

Giesecke T, Williams DA, Harris RE, *et al.* (2003). Subgrouping of fibromyalgia patients on the basis of pressure-pain thresholds and psychological factors. *Arthritis & Rheumatism*, **48**: 2916–22.

Gran TJ (2003). The epidemiology of chronic generalized musculoskeletal pain. *Best Practice & Research Clinical Rheumatology*, **17**: 547–61.

Hughes G, Martinez C, Myon E, *et al.* (2006). The impact of a diagnosis of fibromyalgia on health care resource use by primary care patients in the UK: an observational study based on clinical practice. *Arthritis & Rheumatism*, **54**: 177–83.

Katz RS, Wolfe F, Michaud K (2006). Fibromyalgia diagnosis: a comparison of clinical, survey, and American College of Rheumatology criteria. *Arthritis & Rheumatism*, **54**: 169–76.

Petzke F, Gracely RH, Park KM, *et al.* (2003). What do tender points measure? Influence of distress on 4 measures of tenderness. *Journal of Rheumatology*, **30**: 567–74.

Turk DC, Okifuji A, Sinclair JD, *et al.* (1996). Pain, disability, and physical functioning in subgroups of patients with fibromyalgia. *Journal of Rheumatology*, **23**: 1255–62.

White KP, Speechley M, Harth M, *et al.* (1999). The London fibromyalgia epidemiology study: the prevalence of fibromyalgia syndrome in London, Ontario. *Journal of Rheumatology*, **26**: 1570–6.

Wolfe F, Anderson J, Harkness D, *et al.* (1997). A prospective, longitudinal, multicentre study of service utilization and costs in fibromyalgia. *Arthritis & Rheumatism*, **40**: 1560–70.

Chapter 3

Pathophysiology in fibromyalgia syndrome

Key points

- Pain processing is complex and involves nociception, transmission, modulation, and perception.
- Objective examination using function neuroimaging has demonstrated that pain in patients with fibromyalgia syndrome (FMS) is 'real'.
- Physiological pain is important in protecting us from harm, while maladaptive (pathologic) pain injury is caused by functional abnormality of the nervous system. FMS is characterized by maladaptive pain.
- Sleep study in patients with FMS has confirmed reduced deep quality and increased wakefulness. In healthy volunteers, selective deprivation of non-REM sleep can induce symptoms and hyperalgesic tender sites of FMS.
- Patients with FMS often report experiencing previous stressful or traumatic events. A reduced HPA axis response to stress can contribute to development or worsening of FMS.

In the past, fibromyalgia syndrome (FMS) was often referred to as fibrositis which is a misnomer as -itis implied an inflammatory element. The word 'fibromyalgia' was derived from Latin, meaning a condition of Fibro (fibrous tissue), my (muscles), al (pain), and gia (condition of). Fibromyalgia was most commonly known by the misnomer fibrositis, where Chaitrow asserts that no inflammatory process has ever been found to be part of this disease. Our current understanding of the pathophysiology of FMS is that the disease is a disorder of central pain processing or a syndrome of central sensitivity.

3.1 Understanding pain

Pain is an important physiological mechanism designed to protect us from harm. It warns us of actual or impending danger or damage. Not surprisingly, it is linked to the stress response and reflex withdrawal to protect from further damage or harm. Absence of pain perception as occurs in Charcot joint results in excessive tissue damage and destruction. In the extreme case, such as what occurs in the rare condition hereditary pain indifferent syndrome, the absence of high affinity receptor for nerve growth factor results in the absence of pain sensation. The condition was characterized by multiple Charcot joints, fracture, and deformities. Undoubtedly, pain has an important physiological role both for protection against damage and for encouraging rest to allow repair processes to occur.

Pain can be defined as 'an unpleasant sensory and emotional experience associated with actual or potential tissue damage'. Although it is essentially a sensation, pain has strong cognitive and emotional components. It is interpreted as a suffering resulting in psychological and physiological stress. The latter includes avoidance of motor reflexes, alterations in autonomic output, and increased neuroendocrine response. All of these are intrinsic to the pain experience.

3.1.1 Early theories of pain

The description of pain has a long history dating back to as far as Babylonian times. Early concepts of pain involved the perception that pain was dangerous. Descartes (1664) was the first person to recognize that there was a signalling system involved in the detection of noxious stimuli (Figure 3.1).

He described how, if a subject puts his/her foot in a flame, pain is detected and this information is carried to the organ of perception. The sensory experience of acute pain caused by a stimulus is mediated by the nociceptive system. This system extends from the periphery through the spinal cord, brain stem, and thalamus to the cerebral cortex, where the sensation is perceived. To prevent damage to tissue, we have learned to associate certain categories of stimuli with danger that must be avoided. This is achieved by linking noxious stimuli with a sensation that is intense and unpleasant. The sensation of pain therefore must be strong enough that it demands immediate action. This model of pain was developed further by describing how pain is detected by specific nociceptors which detect tissue damaging stimuli. These stimuli create action potentials which are transmitted via the peripheral nerves to the spinal cord and then to the brain.

The next major breakthrough in the concept of pain was the development of the Gate Control Theory by Melzack and Wall in 1965.

Figure 3.1 Descartes model of pain

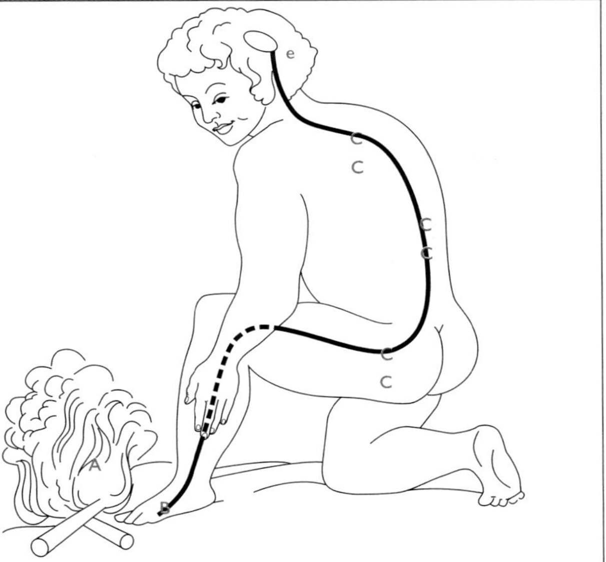

Rene Descartes (1664). L'homme de Rene Descartes. Paris: Charles Angot.

It introduced the idea that the individual had biomedical mechanisms, which could control how pain was understood and appreciated. Much of this is derived from an understanding of the neurological pain pathway where a stimulus from the periphery travels to the brain (Figure 3.2). In addition, there are inhibitory pathways which can control actions. The Gate Control Theory describes how pain can be overridden, 'closing the gate' under certain circumstances. The classic case is that of pain resulting from battleground injuries not being registered until the soldier had been carried from the battleground.

Woolf used the terms adaptive and maladaptive to differentiate physiological pain that protects the organism from injury or promotes healing (adaptive) from pathologic pain due to functional abnormality of the nervous system (maladaptive).

Figure 3.2 The pain pathway

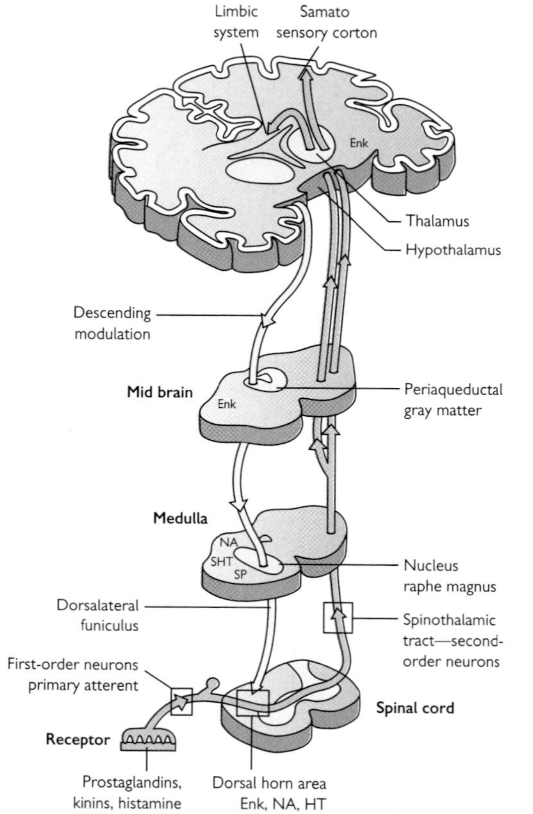

Reprinted from *Rheumatology*, Third edition, Hochberg MC, Silman AJ, Smolen JS, Weinblatt ME, Weisman MH, ISBN 0323024041, published by Mosby (2003), with permission of Elsevier.

3.1.2 **Current theory of normal pain processing**

Pain processing can be divided down into four main parts: nociception, transmission, modulation, and perception.

1. *Nociception*—is the detection of tissue damage or that something is wrong in which a noxious stimulus is detected by a peripheral nociceptor and converted into an electric impulse in the free afferent nerve ending. This is a strongly physical and physiological process and can be inhibited by non-steroidal anti-inflammatory drugs (NSAIDs), opioids, and local anaesthetics.

2. *Transmission*—This is the process whereby nerve impulses are propagated through the peripheral and central nervous system. Sharp pain is conveyed by A-delta (fast) fibres; dull pain is conducted by C (slow) fibres, and tactile sensation is conveyed by A-beta fibres. All these have a lower threshold of stimulation. Transmission can be inhibited by local anaesthetics and alpha-2 agonists.
3. *Modulation*—occurs mainly in the central nervous system, first in the dorsal horn cells of the spinal cord. Excitatory neuropeptides such as substance P, glutamate, and aspartate amplify the pain signals in ascending projection neurons, while endogenous inhibitory descending neurons releasing opioid, serotonin, and noradrenaline dampen the nociceptive response. Local anaesthetics, alpha-2 agonists, opioids, NSAIDs, tricyclic antidepressants, serotonin-selective reuptake inhibitors (SSRIs), and *N*-methyl-D-aspartate (NMDA) receptor antagonists can affect the balance between pain amplification and inhibition.
4. *Perception*—is the cerebral cortical response to nociceptive signals. It relies heavily on the interpretation of the initial stimulus. This process has huge inter-individual variability—a minimal stimulus in some subjects can result in them registering a large amount of pain, but conversely a large stimulus in others can result in no pain being registered. Perception can be inhibited by general anaesthetics, opioids, and alpha-2 agonists.

3.1.2.1 *Nociceptors*

Nociceptors are mostly bare nerve endings which penetrate past the epidermal/dermal junction and are attached to fine fibres. There are two types of nociceptors: polymodal and high threshold mechano-heat receptors.

Alternatively, the nociceptors can be classified biochemically into two main categories:

- NGF dependent nociceptors which account for 70% of receptors. They require NGF for their development and synapse in laminae I and II outer of the spinal cord.
- Glial derived nerve factor dependent nocioceptors constitute the remaining 30% of receptors. They require Glial derived nerve factor for their development and synapse in lamina III inner. It transduces the effect of physical stimulus such as noxious heat.

Until recently, it was thought that nociceptors were only found in the somatic region but not the viscera. However, a recent study showed that distended bladder becomes painful, suggesting that there is a small population of nociceptors in the viscera. In general, visceral pain is less well localized as somatic pain, which may reflect on the density of the nociceptors.

3.1.2.2 *Nerve fibres*

Sensory nerve fibres conduct signals from the nocioceptors to the spinal cord from various parts of the body. There are at least two major types of nerve fibres thought to be responsible for this process:

- *A-delta nerve fibres*: thought to be responsible for 'acute' or 'fast' pain as it carries electrical messages to the spinal cord at approximately 40mph.
- *C-fibres*: thought to be responsible for 'chronic', 'slow', or 'dull pain' and which carry electrical impulses at approximately 3mph.

Some acute injury activates other sensory nerve fibres that conduct even 'faster' than A-delta fibres, which may activate inhibitory pathways in the spinal cord and brain to override some of the pain messages carried by the A-delta and C-fibres.

These physiological pain processes apply in many musculoskeletal diseases where nociceptors detecting pain are present in structures such as synovium, joint capsule, bone, muscles, and ligaments. When nocioceptors are activated, pain signals will be transmitted by special peripheral nerves to the spinal cord and up to the brain. These messages can be overridden by other signals produced by treatments such as massage, heat, or cold packs, transcutaneous nerve stimulation, medications, or even acupuncture.

3.1.2.3 *Spinal cord*

All sensory information enters the spinal cord via the dorsal root. The dorsal horn of the spinal cord has been divided into laminae I–VI, and it is a vital area for sensory processing. Nociceptors synapse via the superficial laminae.

Numerous pain neurotransmitters are present in the spinal cord. Aspartate and glutamate are the main excitatory amino acids produced by the afferent neurons and are probably the most significant molecules in terms of pain transmission. Their activity is modulated by inhibitory neurotransmitters. This activity is post-synaptic as in descending control mechanisms. The overall result depends on the balance between excitatory and inhibitory neurotransmitters.

There are four main inhibitory processes in the spinal cord:

- *Endogenous opioids*: act pre-synaptically to prevent the information from reaching the spinal cord.
- *Afferent inhibition*: non-noxious stimuli reach the brain much faster than the noxious stimuli; therefore 'the gate' can be closed before the pain message reaches the brain.
- *Segmental inhibition*: consists of activation of large afferent fibres subserving epicritic sensation inhibitory neurons and spinothalamic activity. Glycine and amino butyric acid (GABA) are amino acids that function as inhibitory neurotransmitters.

- *Descending inhibition*: several supraspinal structures, including the periaqueductal grey, reticular formation, and nucleus raphe magnus, send fibres down the spinal cord to inhibit pain at the level of the dorsal horn. Axons from these structures act pre-synaptically on the primary afferent neurons and post-synaptically on second-order neurons. These inhibitory pathways utilize neurotransmitters such as noradrenaline and serotonin, on nociceptive neurons in the spinal cord as well as on spinal inhibitory interneurons which store and release opioids. Noradrenaline mediates this action through alpha2 receptors. The endogenous opiate system acts via enkephalins and beta-endorphins. These mainly act pre-synaptically, whereas the exogenous opiates act post-synaptically.

3.1.2.4 *Brain*

Until recently, how the brain perceives pain is poorly understood. In the past, pain was thought of as an extension of the sense of touch. Neuronal signals from the dorsal horn of the spinal cord transmit to the specialized areas of the somatosensory cortex via the thalamus. With the advent of functional neuroimaging using the latest technology such as functional magnetic resonance imaging (fMRI), it has become clear that aside from the somatosensory cortex, many areas of the brain are involved in pain perception. A detailed explanation is beyond the scope of this book. Briefly, there is growing evidence that the parieto-insular cortex is crucial for pain processing in the brain. The area is strongly activated during pain. Lesions in this region can strongly reduce pain perception. Another important area is the caudal part of the anterior cingulate cortex, which has been implicated in the control of motivational behaviours. Activation of this area is linked to perception of the unpleasantness of pain, and is accompanied by activation in several sub-cortical sites, such as the amygdala, cerebellum, and striatum, whilst other areas of the brain such as the rostral anterior cingulate cortex have been implicated in pain modulation/inhibition.

3.1.3 **Maladaptive pain**

Maladaptive pain may be acute or chronic. One of the key features of maladaptive pain is increased sensitivity or hyper-responsiveness. This indicates that pain perception is not 'hard-wired' but 'plastic' and dynamic. This is mediated by changes in the nervous system response (neuroplasticity) at peripheral and central locations.

Hyperalgesia is defined as an increased response to a normally painful stimulus. When a noxious stimulus is applied to an area on the arm, there will be a small area of active tissue hyperalgesia due to the sensitivity of local nociceptors in the skin. Over a period of a few hours, a larger area of secondary hyperalgesia develops. In the case of inflammation, this results from the release of some inflammatory mediators which can reduce nociceptor thresholds. This leads to an increased response to painful stimuli: primary hyperalgesia or peripheral sensitization.

Central sensitization refers to an increase in the excitability of spinal neurons.

Central sensitization may result from several mechanisms:

- *Action potential wind-up*: repeated stimulation of dorsal root afferents including nociceptive C-fibres can elicit a progressive increase in the number of action potentials generated, prolong the duration of the discharge by motoneurons and interneurons even after the afferent C-fibres input has stopped.
- *Receptive field expansion*: dorsal horn neurons increase their receptor field such that adjacent neurons in neighbouring areas become responsive to stimuli whether it is painful or not. This is mediated in part by the activation of NMDA receptors in dorsal horn neurons.
- *Hyperexcitability of flexion responses*: increase flexion reflex ipsilaterally and contralaterally.

Molecules that have been implicated in central sensitization include substance P, CGRP, VIP, cholecystokinin, angiotensin, galanin, glutamate, and aspartate. These substances trigger changes in membrane excitability, leading to increased intracellular calcium concentration. For example, glutamate and aspartate activate the NMDA receptor and resultant intraneuronal elevation of calcium, which stimulates nitric oxide synthase to produce nitric oxide. The latter is a gaseous molecule that diffuses out from the neuron and stimulates the formation of cyclic guanosine monophosphate (cGMP) in neighbouring neurons. Nitric oxide has been implicated in the development of hyperexcitability, resulting in hyperalgesia or allodynia.

3.1.4 **Maladaptive pain in FMS**

A characteristic feature of FMS is hyperalgesia (increasing the response to low-level noxious stimuli) and allodynia (painful response to normally non-noxious stimuli). These are likely to be the result of central sensitization. There are several lines of evidence to suggest that the pain experience of patients with FMS is in part the result of disordered pain processing at a central level.

3.1.4.1 ***Evidence from somatosensory stimulation***

Secondary hyperalgesia, pain elicited from uninjured tissues around the site of pain, was found to be increased in patients with FMS than controls. When electric stimuli was applied to the skin, patients with FMS had reduced pain threshold and pain was noted both distally and proximally to the stimulator, lasting up to 20 minutes after the stimulation was terminated.

Patients with FMS have reduced central inhibitory response. Down-regulation of pain threshold can be demonstrated in normal individuals by subjecting them to repeated skin stimulation. When this was compared in female patients with FMS and age-matched healthy women, concurrent tonic thermal stimuli, at both painful and non-painful levels, significantly increased the pain threshold in the healthy subjects but not in the patients with FMS.

When hypertonic saline was injected into the anterior tibial muscle, patients with FMS experienced a longer duration and a larger area of pain than healthy age-matched controls. Pressure pain and the intra-muscular summation pain threshold were significantly lower in patients with FMS.

3.1.4.2 *Evidence from cerebrospinal fluid*

Substance P

Substance P lowers the threshold of synaptic excitability and sensitizes second-order spinal neurons. Two studies have shown a three-fold increase of substance P in the cerebrospinal fluid (CSF) of patients with FMS compared with controls.

Serotonin

Serotonin is a neurotransmitter implicated in sleep, pain perception, headaches, and mood disorders. It is released by some inhibitory neurons. Lower-than-normal levels of serotonin have been observed in patients with FMS.

Nerve growth factor

Nerve growth fFactor is critical for the differentiation, maintenance, and survival of sensory neurons. It enhances the production of substance P in afferent neurons, increasing the person's sensitivity or awareness to pain. In some studies, nerve growth factor was four times higher in the CSF of patients with FMS than in controls.

3.1.4.3 *Evidence from function neuroimaging*

Functional CNS changes can be demonstrated by several different imaging techniques. It is interesting that chronic pain states have been associated with reduced thalamic blood flow, whereas acute pain increases thalamic blood flow. The reason for this difference is postulated to be a disinhibition of the medial thalamus which results in activation of a limbic network. Mountz *et al.* reported that patients with FMS had a decreased thalamic and caudate blood flow compared with healthy controls on single-photon-emission-computed tomography imaging.

Altered pain processing has also been demonstrated by studies using fMRI where painful pressure stimuli result in increased cerebral blood flow in areas associated with activation by noxious stimuli; and this is exaggerated in patients with FMS at stimulus intensities that are non-noxious in normal individuals, implying that they have reduced pressure pain threshold.

Taken together, there is substantial evidence to suggest that abnormal pain processing is important in the pathophysiology of FMS.

3.2 Sleep

One of the most important advances in the understanding of FMS is the association with sleep disturbance. Most patients with FMS complain of non-restorative sleep. Sleep study in patients with FMS has confirmed that reduced sleep quality is associated with non-dreaming, non-rapid eye movement (non-REM) sleep with interruption by alpha waves. In healthy volunteers, selective deprivation of non-REM sleep can induce symptoms and hyperalgesic tender sites of FMS.

Growth hormone, produced during delta sleep, is involved in tissue repair. Growth hormone also stimulates the production of insulin-like growth factor-1 in the liver. Some studies have found low levels of growth hormone and insulin-like growth factor-1 in patients with FMS. Therefore, disrupted stage 4 (delta) sleep associated with FMS may account for these findings.

3.3 Hypothalamic–pituitary–adrenal axis

Dysfunction of the hypothalamic–pituitary–adrenal (HPA) axis has been implicated in the pathophysiology of FMS. The HPA axis is a critical component of the stress-adaptation response which includes various body processes such as digestion, the immune system, mood, and energy. In a normally functioning system, corticotropin-releasing hormone (CRH) stimulates the anterior pituitary to release adrenocorticotropic hormone (ACTH). ACTH then stimulates the adrenal cortex to produce glucocorticoids, which are powerful mediators of the stress-adaptation response. The normal circadian rhythm for the release of these hormones leads to rapid increase in cortisol level after wakening, reaching a peak within 30–45 minutes. It then gradually falls over the day, rising again in late afternoon. Cortisol levels then fall in late evening, reaching a trough during the middle of the night. Stress induces release of CRH from the hypothalamus is influenced by blood levels of cortisol and by the sleep/wake cycle. Increased production of cortisol mediates responses to stress, allowing the body to attempt countermeasures. However, in excess cortisols can be damaging. Atrophy of the hippocampus in humans and animals exposed to severe stress is believed to be mediated by prolonged exposure to high concentrations of cortisol.

Anatomical connections between brain areas such as the amygdala, hippocampus, and hypothalamus facilitate activation of the HPA axis. Sensory information arriving at the lateral aspect of the amygdala is processed and conveyed to the central nucleus, which projects to several parts of the brain involved in responses to fear. At the hypothalamus, fear-signalling impulses activate both the sympathetic nervous system and the modulating system of the HPA axis. Deficiencies of the hippocampus may reduce the memory resources available to help a body formulate appropriate reactions to stress.

In patients with FMS, a reduced HPA axis response to stress has been demonstrated. The main HPA abnormalities in FMS are as follows:

- Low free cortisol levels in 24-hour urine samples
- Loss of the normal circadian rhythm with elevated evening cortisol level
- Insulin-induced hypoglycaemia associated with an overproduction of pituitary ACTH
- Low levels of growth hormone
- Insufficient adrenal release of glucocorticoids to stimulation by ACTH.

Patients with FMS often report experiencing previous stressful or traumatic event. A reduced HPA axis response to stress can contribute to FMS development or worsening of FMS. The HPA axis is also linked to the autonomic nervous system, which is involved in modulating sleep, mood, pain, and cardiovascular activities (including microcirculation of muscles). This could explain many clinical features and the association of FMS with sympathetic nerve system over activity, although more detailed mechanistic studies will be needed to confine a causative relationship.

Furthermore, patients with FMS frequently complain that pain and tenderness are worse in the morning and experience significant morning stiffness; this is lessened after nights when they have had more restful sleep. Although a cause and effect relationship has not been established, dysfunctioning HPA axis may be an important factor in the pathophysiology of these symptoms in FMS.

The neurotransmitter, serotonin, has a role in regulating the circadian rhythm and the stress-induced stimulation of the HPA axis. This may partly explain the abnormalities of the HPA axis in FM. Alternatively, dysfunction of the HPA axis may exaggerate the effects of abnormal serotonin metabolism, resulting in low serotonin level associated with FMS.

Alternatively, dysfunctional HPA axis has been implicated in the pathophysiology of many disorders including anxiety, depression, post-traumatic stress disorder, chronic fatigue syndrome, sleep disturbances, and irritable bowel syndrome. HPA abnormalities may reflect other comorbidities.

3.4 **Summary**

Although the pathogenesis of FMS is not completely understood, the currently known abnormalities substantiate the proposal that FMS can no longer be considered a subjective pain condition. Somatosensory abnormalities, CSF studies, and functional neuroimaging all lead to a whole body of evidence suggesting that maladaptive pain response is at the core of FMS. Ongoing research will continue to provide a clearer picture of the pathophysiology of this complex syndrome.

Suggested reading

Bennett RM (1998). Disordered growth hormone secretion in fibromyalgia: a review of recent findings and a hypothesized etiology. *Zeitschrift fur Rheumatologie*, **57**: 72–6.

Clauw DJ (1995). The pathogenesis of chronic pain and fatigue syndromes, with special reference to fibromyalgia. *Medical Hypotheses*, **44**: 369–78.

Clauw DJ (2007). Fibromyalgia: update on mechanisms and management. *Journal of Clinical Rheumatology*, Apr; **13**(2): 102–9.

Crofford LJ (1998). The hypothalamic pituitary adrenal stress axis in fibromyalgia and chronic fatigue syndrome. *Zeitschrift fur Rheumatologie*, **57**: 67–71.

Desmeules JA, Cedraschi C, Rapiti E, *et al.* (2003). Neurophysiologic evidence for a central sensitization in patients with fibromyalgia. *Arthritis & Rheumatism*, 1420–9.

Giesecke T, Gracely RH, Williams DA, *et al.* (2005). The relationship between depression, clinical pain, and experimental pain in a chronic pain cohort. *Arthritis & Rheumatism*, **52**: 1577–84.

Gracely RH, Petzke F, Wolf JM, Clauw DJ (2002). Functional magnetic resonance imaging evidence of augmented pain processing in fibromyalgia. *Arthritis & Rheumatism*, **46**: 333–43.

Gracely RH, Geisser ME, Giesecke T, *et al.* (2004). Pain catastrophizing and neural responses to pain among persons with fibromyalgia. *Brain*, **127**: 835–43.

Staud R, Vierck CJ, Cannon RL, *et al.* (2001). Abnormal sensitization and temporal summation of second pain (wind-up) in patients with fibromyalgia syndrome. *Pain*, **91**:165–75.

Chapter 4

Assessing fibromyalgia syndrome

Key points

- A large number of instruments have been used in the assessment of fibromyalgia syndrome (FMS). Some of them have been validated in research in FMS, but there are still significant deficiencies, such as an appropriate tool for assessing cognition.
- Visual analogue scale (VAS) of pain can be used to assess pain intensity in the clinical setting, although there are more sophisticated tools.
- Tenderness/pressure pain threshold can be measured by a simple tool such as a dolorimeter.
- Fibromyalgia Impact Questionnaire (FIQ) is a multi-dimensional validated tool that assesses many major features of the condition.
- Hospital Anxiety and Depression Scale (HADS) is a simple and useful self-completed screening questionnaire for mood disturbances in patients attending routine outpatient clinic. It can be useful in identifying patients with severe depression which needs referral to psychiatrist.
- Using a combination of these assessment methods, sub-groups of patients with FMS could be identified. These could be used to guide treatment regime.

4.1 Introduction

In musculoskeletal diseases, many assessment tools/instruments currently used in routine practice were developed initially for clinical research. As such, they were designed to have the properties to aid understanding of the disease pathophysiology or to determine whether inventions are effective. For routine clinical practice, assessments are often performed to determine disease severity, especially if there are predictors of important outcome and co-morbidities, as well as to identify subsets of patients in whom the result of the assessment helps to inform choice of treatment and subsequent response to therapy. Given these different objectives, not all instruments used in clinical research are suitable for clinical practice. A good assessment tool needs to have certain characteristics. First, it needs to truly measure what it intends to measure. Second, it must be sufficiently specific and also sensitive to change. Third, it should be feasible to carry out the assessment. Hence a valid, sensitive, and specific assessment tool which requires 60 minutes to complete will be feasible in the setting of research but impractical for routine outpatient clinic.

4.2 Assessment tools in FMS

Numerous instruments have been used in clinical trials of FMS. In part, this is due to lack of consensus on what should be measured. Most of these instruments have been developed and validated for use in other conditions, such as other chronic painful diseases, sleep disorders, depression, and anxiety. The only exception is the Fibromyalgia Impact Questionnaire (FIQ), which was developed specifically for FMS, as a tool to assess symptoms of disease, function, and quality of life.

Since FMS is a complex condition with multiple symptoms, determining which components should be assessed is not straightforward. Consequently, a working group on FMS was convened under the auspices of the Outcome Measures in Rheumatology Arthritis Clinical Trials, an organization whose mission is to foster global consensus and developing outcome measurements for clinical trials. Patient focus groups and Expert Delphi process were used by the FMS working group to identify key outcome domains which should be assessed in research. There was a significant agreement by both methods that pain, patient global evaluation of disease, fatigue, quality of life, multidimensional function, sleep, depression, physical function, tenderness, cognition, and anxiety are the most important domains. The exception was stiffness, which was ranked important by patients, but not by physicians/researchers.

4.2.1 Pain

Obviously, pain is the dominant symptom in FMS. Pain has been measured by many instruments. All of them are based on patient reported severity. The commonest and simplest methods are paper-based Visual Analogue Scale (VAS) and Numeric Rating Scale. In clinical trials, there is a need to assess accurately changes in pain intensity over time. The McGill Pain Questionnaire and Brief Pain Inventory are validated questionnaires which have been used extensively in chronic painful conditions. Both have been used in clinical trials of FMS.

4.2.1.1 *VAS and Numeric Rating Scale*

VAS and Numeric Rating Scale often ask patients to rate the average, minimal, and maximal pain intensity during a defined period: 24 hours, last week, or last month. However, the memory of pain intensity is not accurate enough, resulting in significant measurement error. Such recall bias or error could be reduced by using questions that relate to specific activities collected in a diary. Better still, a real-time electronic diary, using alarms to remind patients to score pain severity at fixed times was found to be superior to paper-based method. However, such method may not be feasible in routine clinical practice.

4.2.1.2 *McGill Pain Questionnaire*

The McGill Pain Questionnaire assesses detailed character of the pain experience by letting patients choose appropriate words describing the distinctive aspects of pain and categorize pain into sensory, affective, evaluative, and miscellaneous sensory components. These are then used to calculate a pain rating index. However, it is fairly lengthy with 76 questions in total. A shortened version, Short Form-McGill Pain Questionnaire, has only 15 items in sensory and affective categories that have been validated in FMS and shown to distinguish fibromyalgia pain from other rheumatic conditions.

4.2.1.3 *Brief Pain Inventory*

The Brief Pain Inventory assesses not only the intensity and quality of pain, but also how the impact interferes with activity and, therefore, elements of quality of life. It is a 15-item questionnaire which was developed originally for assessing pain intensity in patients with cancer and how it interferes with the patient's life. Patients are asked to rate the extent that pain interferes with their life on a 0–10 scale across seven domains: general activity, walking, mood, sleep, work, relations with other persons, and enjoyment of life. More recently, it has been used in clinical trials of non-malignant chronic painful conditions, including FMS, in which it has been shown to be feasible and sensitive to change.

4.2.1.4 *Pain Drawing*

Although patients with FMS complain of widespread pain, the extent of pain over the body is not constant. Hence the interest in assessing the location of pain over time. One common method to evaluate this is by pain drawings. Patients are asked to shade the painful areas of their body on mannequins (Figure 4.1). This method has been used not only in assessing efficacy in clinical trials but also in population surveys as a screening tool for patients with FMS. Individuals who shade all four quadrants on the mannequins are deemed to have widespread pain. Interestingly, patients with FMS tend to highlight non-articular areas, while patients with rheumatoid arthritis tend to restrict their score to joint areas.

4.2.2 Tenderness

Intuitively, tenderness may seem to relate to pain. However, spontaneous self-reported pain and stimulus-evoked pain are mechanistically different. The latter is an indication of hyperalgesia and allodynia. Two commonly used methods to assess tenderness in FM are tender point count and dolorimetry.

4.2.2.1 *Tender point count*

Although the number of tender points is part of the American College of Rheumatology (ACR) classification criteria, its role in the assessment of FMS remains unclear. Some researchers have found that tender point count was a crude measure of allodynia to pressure, since it is affected by psychological distress and produced higher score in females.

Others have found that tender point count correlated with pain intensity measured by VAS and neuropathic pain score, but not with anxiety, depression, or somatization; therefore it was argued that it be included as a marker for the severity of neuropathic pain. In many studies, the number of positive fibromyalgia tender points is included as part of disease activity assessment; a more detailed evaluation which includes the severity of the tenderness at each site is included in the

Figure 4.1 Mannequin for pain drawing

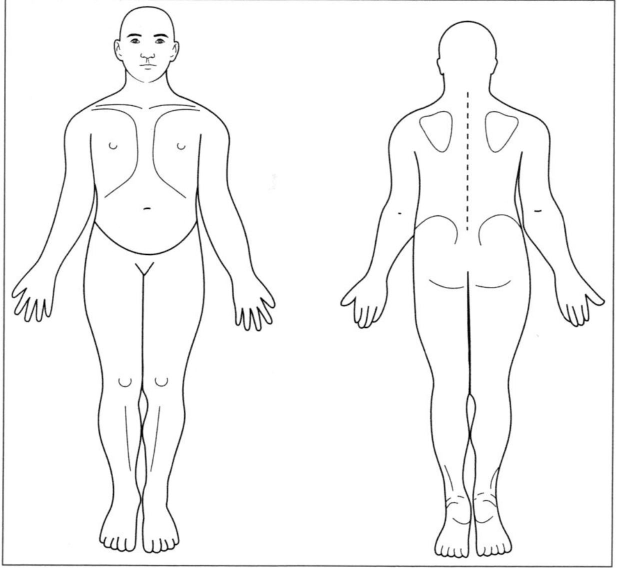

Manual Tender Point Survey. As an outcome measure in clinical trials, tender point count is feasible and sensitive to change.

4.2.2.2 ***Pressure pain threshold measurement***

Pressure algometry measured by a dolorimeter (Figure 4.2) is a semi-objective quantitative method to assess pressure pain threshold. It has been used in clinical trials as well as routine practice. Compared to healthy controls, patients with FMS exhibit lower pressure pain thresholds which are not restricted to the tender points, suggesting generalized allodynia to pressure. However, the exact methodology is not standardized, but some researchers have found that assessments of three-paired tender point sites provide a representative value for the average pressure pain thresholds.

There are numerous methods that have been developed to understand the pathophysiology of pain in fibromyalgia. Most of these are beyond the scope of this book because they are currently not applicable either to clinical trials or to routine practice.

4.2.3 **Fatigue**

Fatigue is a common feature of FMS. Since fatigue is common in many medical illnesses and musculoskeletal conditions, a number of instruments validated in other diseases have been used in clinical trial of FMS. These can be divided into two broad categories: unidimensional and multidimensional. Unidimensional instruments measure intensity without exploring the underlying cause or impact of fatigue.

Figure 4.2 A dolorimeter

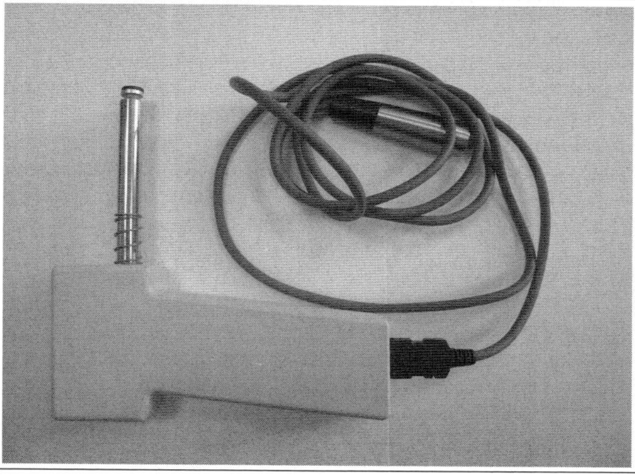

The commonest unidimensional instruments used are VAS, Functional Assessment of Chronic Illness Therapy-Fatigue Scale, and Fatigue Severity Scale. The Functional Assessment of Chronic Illness Therapy Questionnaire is a generic health instrument which has a fatigue domain. The 13-item questionnaire for the fatigue domain has been used extensively in the clinical trial of inflammatory arthritis. The Fatigue Severity Scale was originally developed for multiple sclerosis and systemic lupus erythematosus; in clinical trials of FM, it was sensitive to change.

Multidimensional instruments for measuring fatigue that have been used in clinical trials in FM include Multidimensional Assessment of Fatigue and Multidimensional Fatigue Inventory. The former is a 16-item instrument measuring four dimensions of fatigue: severity, distress, degree of interference in activities of daily living, and timing. The Multidimensional Fatigue Inventory is a 20-item self-report instrument and contains five dimensions: general fatigue, physical fatigue, mental fatigue, reduced motivation, and reduced activity. It was developed initially for assessing fatigue in patients with cancer but has been used in musculoskeletal diseases.

4.2.4 Sleep

Non-refreshed sleep is common and thought to be an important pathological feature in FMS. Objective and detailed evaluation to assess sleep quantity by polysomnography is not feasible for multicentre clinical trial or routine practice. However, they can be used in mechanistic studies.

Commonly, VAS has been used to assess sleep quality anchored by 'sleep is no problem' at one end and 'sleep is a major problem' at the other. Similar scale is used on the 'restedness' domain in the Fibromyalgia Impact Questionnaire (FIQ).

The Medical Outcome Sleep Scale, Pittsburgh Sleep Quality Index, and Jenkins Sleep Questionnaire provide more detailed assessment of both sleep quality and quantity. All have been used in clinical trials in FMS, although they have not been validated against findings from polysomnography study. A 17-item Sleep Assessment Questionnaire has recently been shown to be an excellent screening questionnaire for identifying people with FMS.

4.2.5 Multidimensional function and health-related quality of life

In chronic diseases, curative treatments are unavailable, but many therapies reduce disease severity, improve symptoms and signs, and make patients 'feel better'. Such improvement is usually reflected in physical function, emotional well-being, and participation in family, work, and social life. This is the rationale for measuring generic health status and health-related quality of life. The latter has been defined as those attributes valued by patients and include their resultant comfort or sense of well-being; the extent to which they were able to maintain reasonable physical, emotional, and intellectual function; and the degree to which they retain their ability to participate in valued activities within the family, in the workplace, and in the community. By definition, health-related quality-of-life instruments are multidimensional and hierarchical with measurement of symptoms, function, physical and mental health as well as social, vocational, and social participation. Such instruments can be disease specific or generic. The latter is often used in health economic evaluation as the benefit of different interventions in a wide range of medical conditions can be compared.

4.2.5.1 *Fibromyalgia Impact Questionnaire*

FIQ is a disease-specific 20-item self-report instrument. It is the most commonly used multidimensional disease-specific instrument in FMS. It has eight domains: physical functioning, days well, work, pain, fatigue, morning stiffness, anxiety, and depression. Although the FIQ is a validated instrument and is extensively used in clinical trials, its sensitivity to changing and scaling properties, especially its ability to assess physical function, has been questioned.

4.2.5.2 *Medical Outcomes Short Form-36 Health Survey*

The Short Form-36 (SF-36) is one of the commonest generic health status instrument used in clinical trials. It is a generic health status instrument which has been validated in a broad range of diseases. It has eight domains: physical functioning, role limitations because of physical problems, bodily pain, general health perceptions, energy/vitality, social functioning, role limitations due to emotional problems, and mental health. These can be combined into two summary scores: physical component score and mental component score.

4.2.6 Physical function

Although FMS is associated with significant physical disability leading to high medical and societal cost, there is no validated tool to measure physical disability in FMS, although there is a physical component domain within the FIQ and SF-36 has the physical component score. Similarly, Brief Pain Inventory has a component of physical function in its interference domains. Whether these are adequate assessment of physical function in FMS is unknown.

4.2.6.1 *Health Assessment Questionnaire*

The Health Assessment Questionnaire (HAQ) was developed for musculoskeletal diseases. It includes 20 items assessing eight domains, all of which assess physical functioning. Recently adapted versions of the HAQ have included psychological domains so as to adopt it for assessing a condition such as FMS. Its performance as an outcome measure for FMS has not been fully assessed.

4.2.7 Mood: depression and anxiety

Mood disturbance, depression, and anxiety are common in FMS and an important part of its pathophysiology. Tools used for assessing mood disturbances, depression and anxiety can be broadly divided into two categories: screening and severity assessment.

4.2.7.1 *The MINI International Neuropsychiatric Interview*

The MINI International Neuropsychiatric Interview is a structured diagnostic interview, which is a validated screening tool for an array of psychiatric diagnoses. It has been applied in clinical trials of FMS to exclude patients with certain psychiatric diagnoses. It is probably too extensive for use in routine clinical settings.

4.2.7.2 *Hospital Anxiety and Depression Scale*

The Hospital Anxiety and Depression Scale (HADS) is a self-reported screening questionnaire for assessing depression and anxiety. It consists of 14 questions: 7 for anxiety and 7 for depression. Originally developed for use in hospital medical outpatient clinics, it has been extensively used in primary care setting. It is a useful screening tool but is insufficiently sensitive to measure change.

4.2.7.3 *The Beck Depression Inventory II*

The Beck Depression Inventory (BDI II) is extensively used in psychiatry to assess severity of depression. It is a 21-item questionnaire which has been extensively validated for many medical and psychiatric conditions. Although it is not a screening or a diagnostic tool, it assesses the severity of depression and allows quantification of change over time. Scores of ≤ 9 indicate a patient is not depressed.

4.2.7.4 *Hamilton Depression Rating Scale*

Hamilton Depression Rating Scale is a 21-item questionnaire which is used extensively in the research of depression. The questionnaire is completed by an assessor rating the severity of symptoms associated with depression, including low mood, insomnia, agitation, anxiety, and weight-loss. It has been used in a small number of trials in FM.

4.2.7.5 *State-Trait Anxiety Inventory*

State-Trait Anxiety Inventory (STAI) is a self-report questionnaire with two 20-item scales for measuring state-related and trait-related anxiety. The STAI possesses strong psychometric properties for assessing changes in anxiety, but it has not been validated in FMS.

4.2.8 Cognition

Many patients with FMS complain of cognitive symptoms. They often report trouble in remembering things, process information less efficiently, perform well in demanding jobs, and find complex mental tasks to be very tiring. In the past, there was often controversy on whether the perceived cognitive problems could be demonstrated with objective testing; however, recent evidence showed that objective cognitive deficits can be demonstrated in patients with FMS. Interestingly, the cognitive impairment in patients with FMS may be different from other conditions, including chronic fatigue syndrome.

Currently, the techniques needed to objectively measure changes in cognitive function are not practical in a clinical setting. Therefore, clinical evaluation of cognitive function in FMS must rely on patient self-report. Currently, there are no validated measures for assessing cognitive function in FMS.

4.2.9 **Patient global assessment of disease**

Patient global assessment of disease activity is commonly used in clinical trials of many diseases. In clinical trials of FMS, Patient Global Impression of Change, measured on an 11-point scale, has been used extensively. It is sensitive to change. However, as a measurement of change it is more useful for clinical trial than routine practice where measures of disease activity/status are more helpful.

4.2.10 **Catastrophizing and coping strategy**

Catastrophizing is an attributional behaviour in which pain is characterized as awful, horrible, and unbearable. Catastrophizing appears to play a substantial role in the development of pain chronicity. It predicts the onset of a chronic pain condition from an acute painful event. Catastrophizing was once thought to be a symptom of depression but is now recognized as an independent factor that is only partially associated with depression.

Coping Strategies Questionnaire (CSQ) was first developed as a measure of the strategies utilized by patients to cope with chronic pain, and as a measure of the perceived efficacy of those strategies. The CSQ assesses the use of six cognitive coping strategies (diverting attention, reinterpreting pain sensations, coping self-statements, ignoring pain sensations, praying or hoping, and catastrophizing) and one behavioural coping strategy (increasing behavioural activity). Each strategy subscale is composed of six items, and patients are asked to rate the frequency with which they use each strategy on a seven-point scale.

4.3 **Objective tools**

An area of intensive research is to develop objective tools for the diagnosis and assessment of FMS. Among these, the most promising is functional magnetic resonance imaging (fMRI) and polysomnography. Currently, they are used solely in research; because of cost and feasibility they are not applicable in routine clinical settings.

4.4 Assessments in routine clinical practice

FMS is not a homogeneous condition. Recent research suggests there may be three subgroups according to symptom profile. The first subgroup has patients with moderate levels of anxiety, depression, and catastrophizing, and poor pain control but with the highest pain thresholds and low tenderness. Group two patients are those with high levels of anxiety, depression, and catastrophizing and low pain control and considerable tenderness, whereas Group three patients have low levels of anxiety, depression, and catastrophizing, and good pain control, but with very low pain thresholds and the most tenderness. These subgroups of patients may be expected to respond to different management approaches. Given that these patients may need a different approach to treatment, assessing symptoms pertinent to these patient subgroups is important. The key assessments should include pain severity, tenderness, a screening tool for depression such as HADS, and a coping strategy such as CSQ.

4.5 Summary

A large number of instruments have been used in the assessment of FMS. Some of them have been validated in research in FMS, but there are still significant instruments that are lacking, such as an appropriate tool for assessing cognition. For clinical practice, establishing a core set of assessment will be helpful, but they need to be feasible and validated in the routine practice setting.

Suggested reading

Bennett R (2003). The Fibromyalgia Impact Questionnaire (FIQ): a review of its development, current version, operating characteristics and uses. *Clinical and Experimental Rheumatology*, **23**(5 Suppl 39): S154–62.

Bjelland I, Dahl AA, Haug TT, Neckelmann D (2002). The validity of the Hospital Anxiety and Depression Scale. An updated literature review. *Journal of Psychosomatic Research*, Feb; **52**(2):69–77.

Gendreau M, Hufford MR, Stone AA (2003). Measuring clinical pain in chronic widespread pain: selected methodological issues. *Best Practice & Research Clinical Rheumatology*, **17**: 575–92.

Gracely RH, Grant MA, Giesecke T (2003). Evoked pain measures in fibromyalgia. *Best Practice & Research Clinical Rheumatology*, **17**: 593–609.

Mease P, Arnold LM, Bennett R, *et al.* (2007). Fibromyalgia syndrome. *Journal of Rheumatology*, **34**: 1415–25.

Sinclair D, Starz T, Turk D. The manual tender point survey. National Fibromyalgia Association Web site at: www.fmaware.org/site/News2?page=NewsArticle&id=6263 (october 3rd, 2005).

Chapter 5

Management of fibromyalgia syndrome

Key points

- The major treatment goal in fibromyalgia syndrome (FMS) is to empower the patient to regain control over his/her life, by having a positive attitude, and cope better with the condition. There are evidence-based guidelines such as the EULAR recommendations for the management of FMS which can be used in practice.
- A combination of education, non-pharmacological, and pharmacological therapies is usually needed to achieve this goal.
- New therapies for FMS are emerging, offering hope for better treatment in the future. Although these treatments are not curative, they are important adjuvants helping patients to cope better with pain and improve their quality of life.

5.1 Introduction

One common misconception amongst the medical profession is that no effective treatment exists for fibromyalgia syndrome (FMS). Whilst it is true there is no universal panacea or treatments that are curative, there is evidence from randomized control trials showing the benefit of non-pharmacological and pharmacological therapies.

In order to improve the outcome of FMS, the medical profession must acknowledge the problem. The healthcare burden of FMS is undeniable. The epidemiological study in the United Kingdom showed that in the 8 years preceding the diagnosis of FMS, the healthcare utilization for these patients was high and gradually increasing. Therefore, ignoring the problem will not reduce healthcare cost. Since healthcare utilization decreases following the diagnosis of FMS, it provided strong evidence that constructive diagnosis and management can reduce healthcare cost related to FMS.

5.2 EULAR recommendations

In light of this problem, the European League Against Rheumatism (EULAR) established a task force charged with developing evidence-based recommendations on the management of FMS. The purpose was to produce evidence-based recommendations that would primarily help to inform doctors about the treatments that were available for FMS as well as to give some guidelines on how best to manage patients, given that prognosis is poor and complete remission is unlikely. The task force began its work in 2005 and presented its conclusions in 2006. The recommendations were electronically published in 2007 (Table 5.1). It highlights that effective non-pharmacological and pharmacological treatments for FMS are available. It is hoped that these recommendations will assist practitioners to manage patients with FMS constructively.

5.2.1 Development of EULAR recommendations

Management of FMS requires a multidisciplinary approach. Consequently, a multidisciplinary task force of experts in the field of FMS was convened to produce guidelines for its management.

A systematic review of the literature revealed over 180 clinical trials involving more than 60 different treatments. Data were extracted with predefined criteria. A summary was synthesized and presented to the expert task force. The poorest quality studies were excluded. The inclusion of expert opinion in the formation of these recommendations was important to ensure that a balanced and fair view of treatment options was given. Importantly, a patient representative was included in the task force to make sure that interests and concerns of patients were taken into account.

5.3 General approach to the management of FMS

Management of FMS requires a holistic approach. The diverse symptom profile compounds the individuality of each patient and demands an individualistic approach to management rather than a 'one-size-fits-all' attitude. FMS is not a homogeneous condition. In the previous chapter, subgroups of FM were described. These subgroups of patients would therefore be expected to respond to different management approaches.

Table 5.1 EULAR recommendations for the management of fibromyalgia

Recommendation	Level of evidence	Strength
General		
Full understanding of FM requires comprehensive assessment of pain, function, and psychosocial context. FM should be recognized as a complex and heterogeneous condition where there is abnormal pain processing and other secondary features	IV	D
Optimal treatment requires a multidisciplinary approach with a combination of non-pharmacological and pharmacological treatment modalities tailored according to pain intensity, function, and associated features such as depression, fatigue, and sleep disturbance in discussion with the patient	IV	D
Non-pharmacological management		
Heated pool treatment with or without exercise is effective in FM	IIa	B
Individually tailored exercise programmes including aerobic exercise and strength training can be beneficial to some patients with FM	IIb	C
Cognitive behavioural therapy may be of benefit to some patients with FM.	IV	D
Other therapies such as relaxation, rehabilitation, physiotherapy, and psychological support may be used depending on the needs of the individual patient	IIb	C
Pharmacological management		
Tramadol is recommended for the management of pain in FM. Simple analgesics such as paracetamol and other weak opioids can also be considered in the treatment of FM. Corticosteroids and strong opioids are not recommended	IV IIb	D C
Antidepressants, amitriptyline, fluoxetine, duloxetine, milnacipran, moclobemide, and pirlindole, reduce pain and often improve function; therefore, they are recommended for the treatment of FM	Ib	A
Tropisetron, pramipexole, and pregabalin reduce pain and are recommended for the treatment of FM	Ib	A

Hence the management strategy must be tailor-made according to the primary symptoms of concern to that particular patient, bearing in mind the range of treatments that have been shown to be effective.

In patients with pre-existing or clinically suspected depression, potential suicide risk must be assessed. If considered at risk of suicide, urgent psychiatric referral is needed. If the patient is not at risk, they should still benefit from psychiatric referral, especially if the patient accepts that he/she has significant depression or knows that his/her mood has deteriorated.

Patient education is vital in chronic medical conditions but is even more important in FMS, as anxiety and frustration is common at the time of diagnosis. For many patients, knowing that it is unlikely that FMS symptoms will ever completely resolve, but equally that it is not progressive, helps patients to manage the pain and means that they will be less likely to have unrealistic treatment goals.

5.4 Non-pharmacological treatments

A number of non-pharmacological interventions have been examined in randomized control trials in FMS. These include exercise, cognitive behavioural therapy, homeopathy, physiotherapy, acupuncture, magnetism, dietary alterations, and laser therapy amongst others.

5.4.1 Graded exercise

Exercise is beneficial in FMS, particularly aerobic exercise, but it needs to be tailored to individual patient's physical level. Although pain levels may increase initially, physical function, quality of life, sleep, and fatigue improve with sustained exercise. Patients should be made aware of this so as to alleviate a common concern that exercise could worsen their condition. It is often helpful to advise patients to gradually build up the quantity of exercise.

The volume of literature supporting graded exercise in FMS is substantial. A number of systematic reviews have been published; all of them concluded that exercise is beneficial in FMS. It should be noted that exercise rarely improves pain, and this can in fact be worsened at first. However, physical function, tender point count, aerobic performance, and global well-being all improve with exercise. Research has shown that patients with FMS are equally able to carry out exercise as healthy people, but it needs to be tailored according to each individual. Adherence to an exercise programme is important to long-term success.

Some patients find heated pool-based exercise or hydrotherapy particularly helpful. Buoyancy reduces pressure load from the muscles, and the heated water provides relaxation. Pain relief may only be temporary, but treatment can be maintained long term without any safety concerns. Treatment improves pain, function, and reduces tender point count, although availability of a hydrotherapy pool and cost are limiting factors.

5.4.2 Cognitive behavioural therapy

Cognitive behavioural therapy is often delivered in combination with patient education. It can improve pain and function in some individuals either as sole therapy or in combination with exercise. It may be particularly beneficial if provided early after diagnosis to help patients understand FMS and learn how they themselves can be actively involved in its management. Since a permanent cure is unavailable for FMS, patients have to learn to self-manage by developing effective coping strategies which enable them to remain in control over their own life. Cognitive behavioural therapy may help to improve their long-term prognosis by providing more realistic and positive health beliefs.

5.4.3 Warm water baths and exercise (Balneotherapy)

Warm water relieves and improves pain, function, and mood. Whilst the effects may be short-lived once treatment ceases, the risk of side effects is small. Many patients find that taking warm water bath in the evening reduces pain and helps them get sleep.

5.4.4 Other therapies

A range of dietary interventions have been studied in FMS. There is limited evidence on their effectiveness. Complementary therapies including homeopathic remedies and acupuncture have also been reported in the literature, but the quality of evidence is poor and conflicting; it does not allow firm conclusion and recommendation to be made regarding these therapies.

5.5 Pharmacological treatments

Until recently, there was no licensed treatment for FMS. However, a number of pharmacological interventions have been shown to be efficacious in randomized control trials. In 2007, pregabalin was the first drug approved by the Food and Drug Administration for the treatment of FMS in the United States. Subsequently, duloxetine and milnacipran have received approval by the Food and Drug Administration.

Pharmacological treatment can be useful in combination with the non-pharmacological interventions. However, not all are effective. Non-steroidal anti-inflammatory drugs (NSAIDs) are commonly prescribed for FMS to reduce pain. In clinical trials, NSAIDs appear ineffective and their use in FMS is not recommended.

Intolerance to medication is a well-documented problem in patients with FMS. The frequency of side effects to analgesics, NSAIDs, and tricyclic antidepressants is higher when compared with patients with low back pain and rheumatoid arthritis. The precise cause is unknown. Hypothesis included confusion with symptoms of FMS, 'over-interpretation of sensory experiences', and central sensitization.

5.5.1 **Analgesics**

Tramadol is a weak opioid analgesic that improves pain and function in FMS. It is a centrally acting analgesic which inhibits noradrenaline and serotonin re-uptake whilst also being an agonist for the muopioid receptor. Most commonly reported adverse events include nausea, somnolence, constipation, and dizziness.

Other systemic analgesics have been used in short-term studies including lidocaine, ketamine, and morphine. There is doubt over their efficacy for treating a chronic condition such as FMS. Topical analgesics such as lidocaine and capsaicin are not of benefit in this condition.

5.5.2 **Antidepressants**

Antidepressants are commonly prescribed for FMS. The effects of tricyclic antidepressants, selective serotonin re-uptake inhibitors (SSRIs), dual reuptake inhibitors, mono-amine oxidase inhibitors, and serotonin antagonists in FMS have all been studied in randomized control trials.

5.5.2.1 ***Tricyclic antidepressants***

Tricyclic antidepressants such as amitriptyline are used commonly in the management of patients with FMS. They inhibit serotonin and noradrenaline re-uptake, but also affect glutaminergic neurotransmission by acting on histamine, acetylcholine, and N-Methyl-d-Aspartate (NMDA) channels. Randomized control trials of tricyclic antidepressants, amitriptyline, and cyclobenzaprine in FMS showed that they are effective in reducing pain and improving sleep and fatigue. The beneficial effect is independent of their action on mood, as the doses prescribed are much lower than those that were used for depression. Furthermore, the correlation between improvement in mood and pain is at best moderate. However, the tolerability of tricyclic antidepressant is poor. Adverse effects resulting in withdrawal of treatment are common. Common side effects include somnolence, anticholinergic effect such as dry mouth, gastrointestinal symptoms, and neuro-psychiatric disturbances. Tolerability can be improved by starting at very low doses, such as 10mg of amitriptyline and escalating dose slowly and giving the dose a few hours before bedtime.

5.5.2.2 ***Selective serotonin re-uptake inhibitors***

In general, SSRIs have fewer side effects and are better tolerated than tricyclic antidepressants. Consequently, they are often used in FMS. The SSRIs, fluoxetine, citalopram, and paroxetine, have each been evaluated in randomized, placebo-controlled trials, but results are mixed. In two studies, fluoxetine improved symptoms of FMS, including pain, function, fatigue, and depression. In general, the results of studies of SSRIs in FMS have paralleled the experience in other chronic pain conditions. The newer, 'highly selective' SSRIs, such as citalopram, seem to be less efficacious than the older SSRIs, which have some noradrenergic activity at higher doses.

5.5.2.3 ***Serotonin and noradrenaline re-uptake inhibitors (SNRIs)***

Since, tricyclic antidepressants and high doses of certain SSRIs such as fluoxetine inhibit both the re-uptake of serotonin and noradrenaline, seem more effective than highly selective serotonin re-uptake inhibitors, it led some researchers to hypothesize that dual re-uptake inhibitors may be more beneficial in FMS. Although dual re-uptake inhibitors lack anticholinergic effects, they may have better tolerability and side-effect profile than tricyclic antidepressants.

Clinical trials have suggested that the dual re-uptake inhibitor, venlafaxine, is a pain modulator in neuropathic pain, migraine, and tension headaches. An open-label study of venlafaxine in patients with FMS reported improvement in pain, function, pain threshold, fatigue, and quality of life.

Recently, large randomized control trials of two new dual re-uptake inhibitors, milnacipran and duloxetine, have shown that both are efficacious in the treatment of FMS.

In a placebo-controlled trial of milnacipran, 125 patients with American College of Rheumatology (ACR) criteria defined FMS were randomized to receive either placebo or milnacipran 200mg daily. Dose was gradually escalated over 4 weeks to the target dose. Preliminary endpoint was changed in global pain score at week 12. At the end of the study, pain intensity was reduced by 40% compared with 25% in the placebo-treated patients. A 50% or more reduction in pain intensity was reported by 37% of the milnacipran-treated patients compared with 14% in those receiving placebo. Over 70% of patients reported overall improvement in symptoms compared with only 38% in the placebo group. Anxiety and depression improved by over 40% in the milnacipran-treated patients. Fatigue improved by over 20% and stiffness by over 30%. Physical function and quality of life also improved with treatment. Improvement in pain was independent of effect on mood. The most frequently reported adverse event in milnacipran-treated patient was nausea. Other common side effects include abdominal pain, headache dizziness, and palpitations.

The SNRI, duloxetine, is a licensed treatment for depression and diabetic neuropathic pain. The effect of duloxetine in FMS was examined in a randomized control trial in which 207 patients were assigned to receive duloxetine 60mg twice per day or placebo for 12 weeks. At the end of the trial, patients treated with duloxetine had greater reduction of Brief Pain Inventory average pain severity score than placebo-treated patients (–2 versus –1 on a 0–10 scale), which was statistically significant. Duloxetine-treated patients also had statistically significant superior improvements in the number of tender points, stiffness, physical function, depression, and health-related quality of life than placebo-treated patients. Whether the patient suffered from major depressive disorder at baseline did not relate to improvement in symptoms and pain severity of FMS. Side effects include nausea, headaches, insomnia, constipation, and somnolence.

5.5.3 **Anti-epileptics**

Anti-epileptic drugs such as gabapentin and pregabalin modulate pain perception by increasing inhibitory neurotransmission and blocking calcium and/or sodium channels. Their benefit has been demonstrated in chronic pain conditions such as post-herpetic neuralgia and painful diabetic neuropathy.

Pregabalin, an analogue of gamma-amino butyric acid (GABA) and an α-2-delta agonist, was the first medication to be licensed for the treatment of FMS in the United States. In a placebo-controlled trial, 529 patients with FMS were randomized to receive either placebo, 150, 300, or 450mg/day of pregabalin. Dose was escalated to the target dose over 2 weeks. Patients receiving pregabalin 450mg/day had statistically significantly greater reduction in the severity of pain than placebo-treated patients. There were also significant improvements in sleep quality, fatigue, and global measures of change. The most common side effects were dizziness, somnolence, weight gain, and dry mouth. Pregabalin is approved in the USA at doses of either 300 or 450mg/day.

5.5.4 **Sleep modifiers**

Since poor sleep quality is common in FMS, sedatives/hypnotics are widely prescribed for patients with FMS. Hypnotics such as zolpidem act on benzodiazepine receptors that have been shown to improve sleep and fatigue in patients with FMS. However, they did not improve pain; hence they should be used in combination with other treatments.

Recently, the effect of sodium oxybate in FMS was examined in a randomized control trial. Sodium oxybate is a precursor of GABA which increases slow-wave sleep and growth hormone levels. It is a licensed treatment for narcolepsy. In a phase II randomized control trial, improvement in sleep quality was accompanied by reduction in pain and fatigue.

Pramipexole is a dopamine agonist indicated for treatment of Parkinson's disease. It affects the mesolimbic system, which has a role in sleep control. Results from a randomized placebo-controlled trial showed that it improved pain, fatigue, function, and global well-being. Treatment was well tolerated. However, patients were allowed to continue with current medications at a stable dose. Further randomized control trial evidence will be required to confirm its efficacy in FMS.

5.5.5 Others

Tizanidine is a centrally acting alpha-2 adrenergic agonist which may reduce substance P. In open-label study in FM, it improved sleep and reduced pain. Tropisetron and ondansetron are serotonin 3 receptor antagonists which have shown pain and tender point count improvements in patients with FMS but only in very short-term studies (5–10 days). Further investigation is required to confirm the efficacy of these agents in FMS.

Since the completion of the EULAR recommendations more trials have been published reporting promising treatments for FMS, such as gabapentin, which demonstrated improvements in pain, function, and other symptoms, and paroxetine, which was beneficial for function but not pain. Numerous new studies have equally been published for non-pharmacological interventions which, amongst other additions, add support to the use of cognitive behavioural therapy and related therapies.

5.6 Empowering patients to self-management

In order to improve the prognosis of FMS and reduce its burden on patients, their family healthcare funders, and society, it is vital that the condition is recognized and better understood by patients and clinicians. The major goal is to enable patients to regain control over their life, by having a positive attitude and cope better with the condition. Understanding each patient's need and developing a treatment regimen using a combination of non-pharmacological and pharmacological therapies based on the individual's key clinical manifestations and circumstances are critical to achieving this therapeutic objective. Although management options have been limited in the past, new therapies for FMS are emerging, offering hope for better treatment in the future. Whilst these treatments are not curative, they are important adjuvant helping patients to cope better with pain and improve their quality of life.

Suggested reading

Busch A, Barber KA, Overend TJ, Peloso PM, Bombardier C, Schachter CL (2007). Exercise for treating fibromyalgia syndrome. Cochrane Database of Systematic Reviews. **17**(4): CD003786.

Carville SF, Arendt-Nielsen L, Bliddal H, *et al.* (2008). EULAR evidence based recommendations for the management of fibromyalgia syndrome. *Annals of Rheumatic Disease*, **67**: 536–41.

Crofford LJ and Appleton BE (2000). The treatment of fibromyalgia: a review of clinical trials. *Current Rheumatology Reports*, **2**: 101–3.

Goldenberg DL, Burckhardt C, Crofford L (2004). Management of fibro myalgia syndrome. *Journal of the American Medical Association*, **292**: 2388–95.

Rao SG and Clauw DJ (2004). The management of fibromyalgia. *Drugs Today (BARC)*, **40**: 539–54.

Sim J and Adams N (2002). Systematic review of randomized controlled trials of nonpharmacological interventions for fibromyalgia. *Clinical Journal of Pain*, **18**: 324–36.

Turk DC, Vierck CJ, Scarbrough E, Crofford LJ, Rudin NJ (2008). Fibromyalgia: combining pharmacological and nonpharmacological approaches to treating the person, not just the pain. *Journal of Pain*, **9**: 99–104.

Chapter 6

Quick practical guides

The purpose of this chapter is to provide quick summaries and tips to help clinicians with the diagnosis and management of patients with fibromyalgia syndrome (FMS) in daily practice.

6.1 Diagnosing FMS

6.1.1 Useful practical hints for diagnosing FMS

History

- Ask about site, duration, onset, and severity of pain.
- Ask patients whether they feel tired all the time.
- Ask patients whether they sleep well and whether they feel refreshed in the morning.
- Ask patients whether they feel depressed, anxious, or feel pressurized/stressed at home and at work. In patients with depression, ask whether they have any suicidal thoughts. The presence of the latter will need urgent psychiatric assessment.
- Ask patients whether they have any problem with memory or difficulties with concentration, problem solving, and learning new tasks.
- Ask about the impact of illness on daily life, work, and social relationships.
- Remember to ask the 'red flag' symptoms: unexplained weight changes, fever, and snoring.

Examination

- Conduct general medical examination and assess the number of FM tender points.
- Remember the 'red flag' signs: joint swelling, muscle weakness, abnormal gait, skin rashes, delayed tendon reflexes, lymphadenopathy, and focal neurological signs.

6.1.2 **Tender point count**

1. The thumb pad of the examiner's dominant hand is used to apply pressure to the evaluation sites during the tender-point examination.
2. First, the evaluation site should be located visually. Then, the evaluation site should be pressed perpendicularly for 4s.
3. The site should be pressed only once to avoid sensitization.
4. Four kilograms of pressure should be applied to the site, and it is enough force to blanch the examiner's nail bed.
5. The patient should sit on the examination table for evaluation of the first 14 sites. They should lie on their sides, contralateral to the site to be tested for the greater trochanters, and they should lie on their backs for the knees.
6. The patient should respond with a 'yes' or 'no' if they have any pain at the site being examined.

Figure 6.1 American College of Rheumatology classification criteria for FM: tender point sites

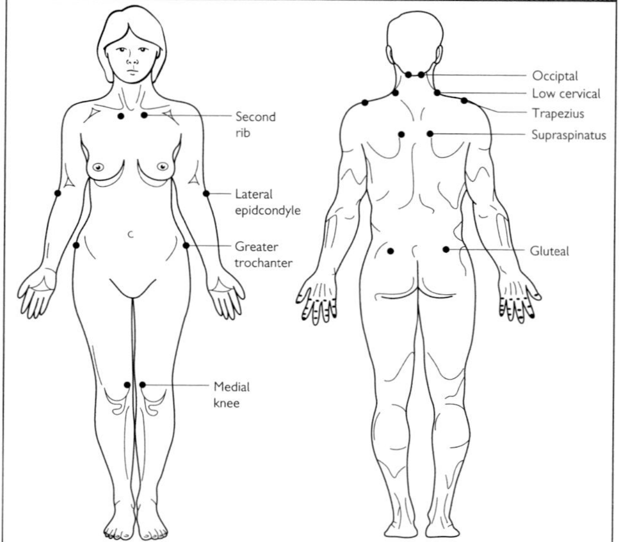

Figure 6.1 is reproduced with permission from Wolfe F, Smythe HA, Yunus MB, *et al.* The American College of Rheumatology 1990 criteria for the classification of fibromyalgia. Report of the multicenter criteria committee. *Arthritis Rheum*, 1990; **33**: 160–72.

Bilateral Sites	Anatomical Location
Occiput	At the nuchal ridge, laterally one-thumb width to the insertion of the suboccipital muscle to the occiput
Low cervical	At the fifth through seventh intertransverse spaces of the cervical spine
Supraspinatus	At the craniomedial border of the scapula at the origin of the supraspinatus
Trapezius	At the upper border of the shoulder in the trapezius muscle, midway from the neck to the shoulder joint
Second rib	In the pectoral muscle at the second costochondral junctions
Lateral epicondyle	Approximately three-finger breadths (2cm) below the lateral epicondyle
Gluteal	In the upper outer quadrant of the gluteus medius
Greater trochanter	Just posterior to the prominence of the greater trochanter at the piriformis insertion
Medial knee	At the medial fat pad proximal to the joint line

6.2 Assessment of pain

6.2.1 Pain drawing

Instructions: Use a pencil or pen to mark darkly on the body diagrams the locations of your pain during the last week.

Figure 6.2 Mannequin for pain drawing

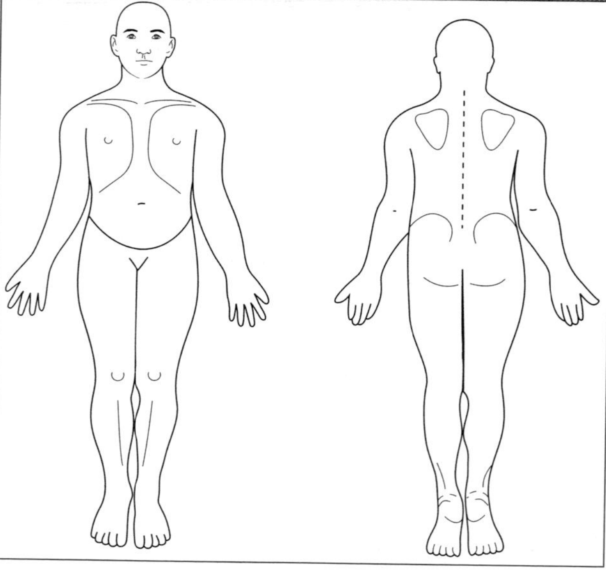

6.2.2 Visual Analogue Scale (VAS) of pain

Figure 6.3 Visual analogue scale of pain

How severe is your pain now?

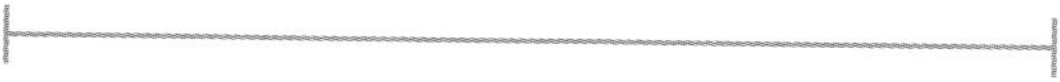

No pain Worst possible pain

Reprinted from *The Lancet*, Huskisson EC (1974). Measurement of pain. *The Lancet*, **304**: 1127–31, Copyright (1974), with permission of Elsevier.

6.3 Assessing mood: Hospital Anxiety and Depression Scale (HADS)

Figure 6.4 Fibromyalgia impact questionnaire

Fibromyalgia impact questionnaire (FIQ)

Last name: First name: Age: Todays date:

Duration of FM symptoms (years): Years since diagnosis of FM:

Directions: For questions 1 through 11, please check the number that best describes how you did overall for the *past week*. If you don't normally do something that is asked, place an 'X' in the 'Not Applicable' box.

Were you able to:	Always	Most	Occasionally	Never	Not Applicable
1. Do shopping?	☐ 0	☐ 1	☐ 2	☐ 3	☐ 4
2. Do laundry with a washer and dryer?	☐ 0	☐ 1	☐ 2	☐ 3	☐ 4
3. Prepare meals?	☐ 0	☐ 1	☐ 2	☐ 3	☐ 4
4. Wash dishes/cooking utensils by hand?	☐ 0	☐ 1	☐ 2	☐ 3	☐ 4
5. Vacuum a rug?	☐ 0	☐ 1	☐ 2	☐ 3	☐ 4
6. Make beds?	☐ 0	☐ 1	☐ 2	☐ 3	☐ 4
7. Walk several blocks?	☐ 0	☐ 1	☐ 2	☐ 3	☐ 4
8. Visit friends or relatives?	☐ 0	☐ 1	☐ 2	☐ 3	☐ 4
9. Do yard work?	☐ 0	☐ 1	☐ 2	☐ 3	☐ 4
10. Drive a car?	☐ 0	☐ 1	☐ 2	☐ 3	☐ 4
11. Climb stairs?	☐ 0	☐ 1	☐ 2	☐ 3	☐ 4
Sub-total scores (*for internal use only*)	☐	☐	☐	☐	☐
Total score (*for internal use only*)	☐				

12. Of the 7 days in the past week, how many days did you feel good? — Score ☐

☐ 0 ☐ 1 ☐ 2 ☐ 3 ☐ 4 ☐ 5 ☐ 6 ☐ 7

13. How many days last week did you miss work, including housework, because of fibromyalgia? — Score ☐

☐ 0 ☐ 1 ☐ 2 ☐ 3 ☐ 4 ☐ 5 ☐ 6 ☐ 7

Directions: For the remaining items, mark the point on the line that best indicates how you felt overall for the past week.

(for internal use only)

14. When you worked how much did pain or other symptoms of your fibromyalgia interfere with your ability to do your work, including housework?

No problem with work |————————| Great difficulty with work — ☐ Score

15. How bad has your pain been?

No pain |————————| Very severe pain — ☐ Score

16. How tired have you been?

No tiredness |————————| Very tired — ☐ Score

17. How have you felt when you get up in the morning?

Awoke well rested |————————| Awoke very tired — ☐ Score

18. How bad has your stiffness been?

No stiffness |————————| Very stiff — ☐ Score

19. How nervous or anxious have you felt?

Not anxious |————————| Very anxious — ☐ Score

20. How depressed or blue have you felt?

Not depressed |————————| Very depressed — ☐ Score

☐ **Sub-total**

☐ **FIQ total**

6.4 Quick guide to management

6.4.1 Quick tips

Many doctors feel diffident in managing patients with FMS. The reasons include a lack of understanding of the underlying pathophysiology, the plethora of symptoms, and a misconception that nothing can be done. This often results in a negative consultation, which is frustrating for both patient and doctor. Here are a few key tips:

1. Be a good listener.
2. Assess patient for severity of pain, tenderness, depression and anxiety, and coping if possible using self-report forms and questionnaires.
3. Do not assume that depression is the basis of fibromyalgia syndrome in all patients. In fact, not all patients are depressed. It is easy to confuse psychosocial stress with depression.
4. In patients with pre-existing or HADS positive or clinically suspected moderate to severe depression, assess for suicide risk. If considered at risk, urgent psychiatric referral is needed. If the patient is not at risk, they should still benefit from psychiatric referral, especially, if the patient accepts he/she has significant depression or knows his/her mood has deteriorated.
5. Although pain is a subjective symptom and cannot be seen, research has shown that these patients are not malingerers. When they complain of pain, that is what their brain is telling them. It is important not to cast doubt on their complaint.
6. Be constructive and explain the nature, prognosis, and treatments available to the patient. Reassure them and discuss treatment strategy.
7. Non-pharmacological interventions are very important. Highlight what patients can do for themselves: warm water bath and graded exercise. Warn patients that pain may worsen transiently when starting exercise but that it should be persevered. Consider cognitive behavioural therapy, relaxation, rehabilitation, physiotherapy, and psychological support which may be used depending on the needs of the individual patient.
8. Pharmacological treatments as recommended by the European League Against Rheumatism (EULAR) recommendations may be a useful adjunct and should be considered. Choice will depend on clinical manifestations.
9. 'Start slow and go slow' is the motto for using medications. Patients with FMS are often very sensitive to side effects from treatment. In many instances, it may be difficult to separate symptoms of FMS from the side effects of treatment. There are

also studies which show that FM patients are more sensitive to treatment side effects. So start on the lowest dose and gradually titrate it upwards.

10. Explain to the patients that the maximum benefit for pain modification treatment such as the antidepressants may take several weeks to exert its maximum effect. Many patients think such treatments are painkillers and expect them to work immediately. If this is not explained, they often give up treatment because they do not respond after a few days.
11. It is vital patients have a realistic expectation from medications. They are not a cure for FMS. On their own it is not the whole answer. Patients must not ignore the non-pharmacological intervention.
12. Do NOT advise the patients to avoid all activities and rest all the time.
13. Work with patients to develop treatment goals and a self-management strategy.

6.5 A practical self-help guide for patients

Here are some practical tips that many patients find helpful.

6.5.1 Patient education

6.5.1.1 *Leaflets*

- FM information pack from Fibromyalgia Association UK
- ARC patient information leaflet on FM.

6.5.2 Patient support groups

- Fibromyalgia Association UK

6.5.3 Useful websites

- www.fibromyalgia-associationuk.org
- www.arc.org.uk

6.5.4 Warm water bath

Many patients find warm water soothing and relaxing. Having warm baths in the morning and evening often helps to start the day and for many patients to sleep better at night.

6.5.5 Exercise

Do not be afraid of exercise. Many patients avoid exercise because their muscles are more painful afterwards. Aching after exercise is normal. Exercise does not cause more damage in FMS. Start gradually and tend to build up the amount of exercise you do gradually. If you have not done exercise for some time, your muscles may ache more. Get advice from your doctor, physiotherapists, or advisor from fitness centre to give you advice on how to build up your exercise.

Try exercise in the evening and take a warm bath afterwards. Many patients find it also helps them to sleep better.

6.5.6 Sleep

If the quality of sleep is poor, you don't feel refreshed in the morning and your partner complains about your snoring, you should tell your doctor. Your doctor may need to refer you to a specialist to see whether you have a specific illness 'sleep apnoea syndrome'.

6.5.7 Mood

Depression, anxiety, and stress can all aggravate FMS. Some patients suffer from depression for many years before they develop FMS. They often notice that depression and anxiety make pain, fatigue, and sleep worse. It is important to discuss this with your doctor especially if it is very bad; you may need additional help from psychiatrist and psychologist. Although depression is not the main cause of FMS, it may be difficult to reduce pain without improving mood in patients who have severe depression.

6.5.8 Dealing with stress

Stress can worsen FMS. Identify areas of life which are stressful; taking measures to reduce stress at work and in the family can be very helpful. Your doctor may provide a letter to explain the nature of FM to your employer. It is good for patients with FMS to work. It improves overall quality of life. The key is to find ways to adapt and reduce excessive stress. Cognitive behavioural therapy can be helpful in developing realistic achievable goal.

6.5.9 Living and coping with FMS

Like many patients with chronic medical illnesses, finding ways to cope is very important. Many patients with FMS feel frustrated and pessimistic. It is important to accept that FMS is a chronic illness; there is no universal panacea. However, treatment can reduce severity of symptoms, allowing patients to regain control over their life.

6.6 When to investigate

It is important not to over investigate. Incidental non-clinical significant findings can cause unnecessary anxiety.

Here are a few suggestions on when to investigate:

1. The presence of objective physical signs.
2. New symptoms when all other aspects of FMS are stable.
3. Unexpected significant weight loss or gain.
4. Fever.
5. When a symptom is very persistent and worsening.

6.7 Summary

It is important to diagnose and manage FMS positively. The key word is to regain control both for the doctor and the patient.

Chapter 7

Case studies

7.1 Case 1: A typical case of fibromyalgia syndrome (FMS)

A 50-year-old environmental manager has developed severe pain over the right costochondral area over the last 18 months. The pain is present especially during the daytime. She has no nocturnal symptoms and has no problem in the morning. She finds that stress aggravates her problem. In addition, she also has pain affecting her arms, legs, back, and neck. These tend to be mechanical; worsened by movement and relieved by rest. She has early morning stiffness that lasts all day. Her joints feel swollen all the time. She admits to sleeping poorly and has occasional paraesthesia and numbness in her hands. Her weight has been steady. Her only current medication is hormone replacement therapy (HRT), which she takes to control mood swings.

On examination, her joints appear normal. There was no detectable synovitis. She has multiple fibromyalgic tender points.

7.1.1 Investigations

Full blood count (FBC), biochemistry, erythrocyte sedimentation rate (ESR), and C-reacting protein (CRP) are normal. Rheumatoid factor (RF) is negative. Anti-nuclear antibody is present at a titre of 1:20. Other auto-antibody tests are negative. Thyroid function tests are normal.

7.1.2 Learning points

- Many patients with fibromyalgia (FM) complain of joints feeling swollen and have prolonged early morning stiffness. This may be confused with inflammatory arthritis.
- Non-restorative sleep is common in FM.
- It is important to enquire about depression.
- It is important to enquire about work and family situation. Whether the patients are under any stress.
- The role of investigations in FMS should be discussed.

7.2 Case 2: Secondary FMS

An 18-year-old woman suffers from juvenile chronic arthritis since the age of 13. Initially she developed a sudden onset of pain in several joints including the ankles, knees, feet, hands, elbows, shoulders, and neck. Swelling has been noticed particularly in the hands and elbows with early morning stiffness lasting 1 hour. The patient also describes locking of the left elbow. The patient was previously treated with methotrexate and her condition improved initially. Her condition worsened 3 years ago with more aches and pains in her joints. She suffers from widespread muscular pain; cramps in the legs, and to a lesser extent in the hands, particularly at night; fatigue; non-refreshing sleep; migraine; stomach pain; numbness in the hands and feet; and pain in the loin. She has an episode of chest pain which is not related to exertion. Past medical history includes migraine, asthma, irritable bowel syndrome, and urinary frequency.

Physical examination revealed a number of tender joints, including feet, hands, ankles, knees, wrists, elbows, and shoulders. None of the joints was swollen. FM tender points were positive 12/18.

7.2.1 Investigations

- FBC and Biochemistry was normal
- ESR: 11mm/hr
- CRP: negative.

Methotrexate dose was escalated but patient did not respond. She complained methotrexate made her dizzy and sick. She wanted to stop methotrexate.

7.2.2 Learning points

- Secondary FMS is not uncommon in patients with inflammatory arthritis.
- It should be suspected in patients with a lot of tenderness or tender joints but no synovitis and no acute phase response.
- Patients with FMS are more likely to complain of side effects from medications.
- These 'side effects' are not easily distinguishable from symptoms of FMS causing confusion.
- Careful evaluation and discussion are needed regarding stopping what might have been effective treatment for the inflammatory condition.

7.3 Case 3: Confusion with inflammatory arthritis

A 34-year-old care worker for disabled people had an approximately 5-month history of pain and swelling in the small finger joints right elbow, both hips, and knees. She suffered from pain all the time, which was aggravated by activities such as driving or opening jars. It sometimes woke her at night. She had early morning stiffness lasting almost all day. Aside from pain, fatigue was a major problem.

The patient did not complain of skin rash, weight change, Raynaud's phenomenon, or neurological symptoms. Her past medical history included gestational diabetes, lichen sclerosis, migraine, dyspepsia, and long-standing mechanical knee pain.

The patient was taking ibuprofen 400mg up to six tablets per day, but found it of limited efficacy. In contrast, felbinac gel was helpful.

On examination, skin and nails were normal. Neither nodule nor lymph node was present. Some joints were tender without any evidence of synovial joint swelling. Fifteen out of eighteen FM tender points were present. The rest of the examination was unremarkable.

7.3.1 Investigations

Negative or normal ESR, CRP, blood count, RF, auto-antibodies, liver function tests, and renal function tests. Radiographs of her hands and feet were normal.

7.3.2 Learning points

- In some cases, differentiating FMS from viral-induced inflammatory arthritis may be difficult, as patients may complain of prolonged early morning stiffness and joint swelling.
- While many patients with FMS may complain of swollen joints, objective evidence of synovitis is often absent.

7.4 Case 4: Overlap with chronic fatigue syndrome

A 45-year-old writer went abroad for a holiday and developed an episode of viral illness of 2 weeks duration characterized by fever, malaise, sore throat, headache, and dry cough. At the time she also experienced generalized muscle pain and fatigue. She was admitted to hospital for investigation but no abnormality was found. Her fever settled and her general condition improved. However, she developed pain in her hands, shoulders, hips, knees neck, and lower back which was constant and aggravated by physical activities. Aside from pain, fatigue was a major problem. She described attacks of severe fatigue which left her completely washed out. She had to give up work and found household chores impossible. Her mood was low because of the persistent pain.

The patient had no other complains. Her past medical history included an episode of depression after the death of her mother. She took paracetamol for the pain, but it was ineffective.

General medical examination was normal. No lymph node was palpable. Joints were tender but not swollen. Eighteen FM tender points were present.

7.4.1 **Investigations**

Results of blood tests were normal.

7.4.2 **Learning points**

- FMS may overlap with chronic fatigue syndrome.
- Some patients complain of a viral infection before disease and may have been extensively investigated for persistent infection.

7.5 Case 5: Chronic localized pain and FMS

A 63-year-old retired cleaner to our clinic presented with long-standing mechanical low back pain with periodical flares over the past 10 years. Each flare lasted 4–6 weeks. Attacks occurred approximately once every 2 months. Although in between attacks she experienced dull ache in her lower back, during these flares, she found it difficult to walk. Bending, prolonged standing, and coughing all aggravated the pain. There was also a history of mechanical pain in the right knee and hip which came on after walking for 15–20 minutes. Finally, she also suffered from fairly regular attacks of pain in the neck for which she had to consult an osteopath. Otherwise, the patient felt well in herself, but her current complaints include cataracts, paraesthesia in the hands and feet, as well as a 'funny feeling' in the stomach with recent onset of vomiting. Over the last year, her symptoms had got worse. It had become more diffuse throughout her body. It was present virtually all the time. She felt tired and slept poorly. Finding a good position to sleep was difficult.

Physical examination revealed reduced flexion in both knees. Right knee was particularly painful, and mild crepitus could be detected. There was tenderness over the lumbar spine, mainly over L5. There was also tenderness over the iliac crest bilaterally. Both flexion and, to a lesser extent, extension of the lumbar spine were painful. Straight leg raising was 80° on the left and 70° on the right with negative sciatic and femoral nerve stretch tests. There were no abnormal neurological signs, and tests for carpal tunnel syndrome were negative. The cervical spine showed restricted range of motion that was painful. Again, there was no evidence of referred pain or neurological sign. Eleven out of eighteen FM tender points were present.

7.5.1 **Investigations**

Results of blood tests were normal. Radiograph of her lumbar spine showed reduced disc space at L4/5 and L5/S1. Her neck X-ray showed degenerative disease with osteophytes and reduced disc space at C5/6. Her knee and hip x-rays showed mild reduction in joint space but were otherwise normal. Magnetic Resonance Imaging (MRI) scan of her neck and lower back only confirmed results of plain radiograph without any evidence of disc prolapse or nerve entrapment.

7.5.2 **Learning points**

- FMS may sometime develop in patients with chronic localized musculoskeletal pain such as osteoarthritis, neck or low back pain.
- It has been postulated that in these patients 'sensory spreading' from central sensitization may be the underlying pathophysiological process.

7.6 **Case 6: A subtype of FMS (low levels of depression and anxiety, normal cognition, tenderness)**

A 35-year-old police officer doing mainly clerical work complains of multiple joint pain affecting mainly the neck, shoulder girdle, lower back, and legs for 5 years. There is significant stiffness in all joints. Her symptoms tend to be aggravated by factors such as stress, cold weather, protracted walking, and climbing stairs, whereas alleviating factors are relaxing activities such as playing chess and rest and comfortable position. In spite of this, the patient usually has significant pain at night, especially turning over in bed. She sleeps poorly at night. She finds it difficult to get to sleep and often wakes up early in the morning. She never feels refreshed in the morning and is tired all the time. The low back pain is of a dull aching type with superimposed episodes of sharp pain, and these are referred to the thighs. She sometimes has paraesthesia in the legs and previously in the feet but no numbness. Walking distance is limited because of shortness of breath and joint pain as well.

She also suffered from severe neck pain, which radiated to the back of her head and triggered off severe headache. She had a long history of suffering from headache, which was investigated extensively, including repeated MRI scans by a neurologist. No abnormality was found and she was told that the headache was atypical migraine.

She lives with her husband and two children in a house, which has a lot of stairs. There is a lot of pressure at work and she has noticed that pain was worse when her stress level was high. Her line manager was neither understanding nor sympathetic. She told her that she had been taking too much sick leave and she looked well to her anyway. Although it was difficult, she has continued working.

At times she has felt depressed and finds it difficult to cope during bad periods. However, her husband has been very supportive and it made a lot of difference. After taking a 2-week holiday, she was feeling much better.

On examination there was no evidence of synovitis in the peripheral joints, skin rash, or skin nodules. She has restricted active range of motion of the cervical spine, with approximately normal passive range of motion. She had 11 out of 18 fibromyalgic tender points. Flexion of the lumbar spine was slightly reduced because of pain.

7.6.1 Investigations

Her blood tests and x-rays were normal. Using the Hospital Anxiety and Depression Scale (HADS) Questionnaire, it was found that she has mild depression and anxiety.

7.6.2 Learning points

- A common subtype of FMS is represented by patients who have pain but only a few tender points, although sufficient in number to fulfil the American College of Rheumatology (ACR) criteria. They often have mild depression and anxiety, but they are coping with the pain.
- Anti depressants may be particularly helpful.

7.7 Case 7: A subtype of FMS (high level of tenderness and depression)

A 52-year-old retired author presented with long-standing generalized pain in her joints and muscles over the past 15 years. The patient feels her symptoms started when she was attacked by robbers and was hit at the back of the head and kicked repeatedly. Recently, the pattern of pain has changed. It is now more severe, frequently severe at night. All her joints are affected, including her neck and back. She can not do anything. The patient is in considerable pain in the evening when sitting down. Any movement tends to aggravate the pain. She can not even hold a pen or a cup. She cannot get comfortable in bed. Pain is so severe that she cannot get to sleep. She only sleeps 2–3 hours at night. Consequently, she is completely washed out. Her appetite is poor. She has a history of suffering from depression. Her mood is very low, often tearful, and she feels she cannot cope anymore. She is stiff all day and cannot understand clearly why she seems to be in a 'fog' all the time. It is impossible for her to write, and her memory is poor. She suffers from dizziness, palpitation, and excessive swelling. She had two blackouts and was admitted to hospital through the Accident and

Emergency Department. She has extensive investigations organized by cardiologists and neurologists; MRI scan, echocardiography, 24-hour ECGs were all normal. She is very concerned because no cause has been found for these blackouts. Her hands and feet suffer from attacks of numbness and paraesthesia.

There is also no history of bowel problems: dyspepsia, diarrhoea, and abdominal pain. She is currently being investigated by an urologist for frequent urination and dysuria, but her repeat urinary cultures are normal.

She is given different kinds of medicines, but they all make her sick. She gets side effects from all of them and they are not helpful in anyway. She cannot remember the names of these medications.

In the middle of the consultation, she bursts out in tears and claims she cannot cope with all these problems anymore.

Examination revealed absence of synovitis, skin rash, and lymphadenopathy. Her chest was clear and there were no abnormal heart sounds. Neurological examination was normal. Eighteen FM tender points were present. She was tender seemingly all over. It was difficult to examine the patient as she appeared very tense. Back and neck movements were restricted in all directions because of pain.

7.7.1 **Investigations**

FBC, biochemistry, RF, ESR, and CRP were normal or negative. Antinuclear antibody was present at a titre of 1/20, but anti-DNA-ds antibodies were absent. X-ray of the cervical, lumbar spine, hands, and feet revealed minor degenerative changes but no other abnormalities. Nerve conduction study was normal. Twelve-lead electrocardiogram (ECG), chest x-ray echocardiography, 24-hour ECG, and MRI scans of the brain and spine were all normal.

7.7.2 **Learning points**

- This type of FM patient is commonly seen in secondary and tertiary care. They are characterized by high number of tender points, tenderness, high level of anxiety and depression, disturbed cognition, and loss of control or catastrophizing, defined as having a very negative and pessimistic view of their pain. They are polysymptomatic, and sympathetic symptoms are common.
- Low titre of auto-antibodies such as anti-nuclear antibody are found in normal individuals; on its own is not diagnostic for autoimmune diseases.
- Many patients with FMS gave a history of significant depression pre-dating the development of chronic widespread pain. Often these patients have a depression-driven FM. They should be referred to a psychiatric team for management.

- In patients with significant depression and expressing hopelessness, it is important to enquire about suicidal thoughts. Those patients with suicidal thoughts should be referred for urgent psychiatric assessment.
- This patient subtype has the worse prognosis.

7.8 Case 8: A subtype of FMS (tender, no negative psychological or cognitive factors)

A 42-year-old manager has suffered from widespread pain in her joints and muscle for 20 years. She could not remember how it started but seemed to have suffered from it as far as she could recall. There was no specific precipitating event nor aggravating or relieving factor. There is significant variation in severity from day to day. She feels tired but she puts this down to either being very busy at work or sleeping poorly. Although she sleeps for 8 hours per night, she does not feel refreshed in the morning. The pain has got worse recently. She and her husband have noticed that even light touch can cause pain. They have become alarmed and therefore seek medical advice. Otherwise her general health is good. Mood is normal, and there is no history of cognition problem.

Examination revealed 14 fibromyalgic tender points, but general medical examination was normal. Light pressure was sufficient to elicit pain.

7.8.1 Investigations

FBC and biochemistry were normal. The patient completed the Hospital Anxiety and Depression Questionnaire, which was normal.

7.8.2 Learning points

- This patient subtype has a good prognosis.
- Patients with significant functional impairment should be encouraged to exercise.
- Cognitive behavioural therapy may be helpful.

Index